Preventive Nutrition
and Society

Proceedings of the British Nutrition Foundation
Second Annual Conference held at
The Royal Society, July 1 – 2, 1980

Preventive Nutrition and Society

edited by

M. R. Turner

British Nutrition Foundation
London, England

1981

Academic Press

A Subsidiary of Harcourt Brace Jovanovich, Publishers
LONDON · NEW YORK · TORONTO · SYDNEY · SAN FRANCISCO

ACADEMIC PRESS INC. (LONDON) LTD.
24/28 Oval Road
London NW1 7DX

United States Edition published by
ACADEMIC PRESS INC.
111 Fifth Avenue
New York, New York 10003

British Library Cataloguing in Publication Data

Preventive nutrition and society
   1. Medicine, Preventive   2. Nutrition
   I. Turner, M. R.
   614.5′93′9   RA601

   ISBN 0 – 12 – 704450 – 7

LCCN 81 – 66688

Filmset by Reproduction Drawings Ltd., Sutton, Surrey
and printed in Great Britain by T. J. Press (Padstow) Ltd., Padstow, Cornwall

Contributors

Eva Alberman
Professor, Department of Clinical Epidemiology, The London Hospital Medical College, Turner Street, London E1 2AD

Arnold E. Bender
Professor, Department of Nutrition, Queen Elizabeth College, Atkins Building, Campden Hill, London W8 7AH

Timothy V. N. Fortescue
Secretary-General, Food and Drink Industries Council, 25 Victoria Street, London SW1H 0EX

W. Phillip T. James
Assistant Director, MRC Dunn Clinical Nutrition Centre, Addenbrooke's Hospital, Cambridge CB2 1QE

William A. Laing
Consultant Economist, 62 Croftdown Road, London NW5 1EN

Judith M. Lannon
Director and Head of Creative Research, J. Walter Thompson Company Ltd., 40 Berkeley Square, London W1X 6AD

Douglas S. Leathar
Director, Advertising Research Unit, Department of Marketing, University of Strathclyde, Stenhouse Building, 173 Cathedral Street, Glasgow G4 0RQ

John C. McKenzie
Principal, Ilkley College, Wells Road, Ilkley, West Yorkshire LS29 9RD

Jean W. Marr
Dietitian and Honorary Lecturer, Department of Clinical Epidemiology and Social Medicine, Royal Free Hospital School

of Medicine, The Royal Free Hospital, 21 Pond Street, London NW3 2PN

Malcolm N. Naylor

Professor, Department of Periodontology, Guy's Hospital, London Bridge, London SE1 9RT

Michael N. Nelson

Research Officer, MRC Dunn Nutrition Unit, Cambridge. Present address: MRC Environmental Epidemiology Unit, South Academic Block, Southampton General Hospital, Southampton SO9 4XY

Alison Paul

Scientific Officer, MRC Dunn Nutrition Unit, Milton Road, Cambridge CB4 1XJ

Sylvia Robert-Sargeant

Education Director, British Nutrition Foundation, 15 Belgrave Square, London SW1X 8PS

Antony J. Smith

Deputy Editor, British Medical Journal, Tavistock Square, London WC1H 9JR

Ruth Squire

Headteacher, Ashley Down Infants' School, Downend Road, Bristol BS7 9PE

Angus M. Thomson

Director (Retired), MRC Reproduction and Growth Unit, Princess Mary Maternity Hospital, Great North Road, Newcastle upon Tyne NE2 3BD

Preface

The developed world has emerged only recently from a history of poverty, food shortage, poor sanitation and a low level of health care—the situation still faced by less-developed countries today. In such conditions, infectious diseases predominate as causes of ill health and death.

With rising affluence the food supply, sanitation and health-care improve. As a consequence, infectious diseases become less prevalent, and when they do occur good facilities exist for their treatment. In affluent societies, therefore, the pattern of disease has changed and the major hazard to health is now from diseases of an inappropriate life-style. The magnitude of the health problem remains large. In Britain, disease and death in infancy and childhood are substantially less than 100 years ago, but the morbidity and mortality rates of adults below retirement age remain at an unacceptably high level.

The many so-called "diseases of affluence" in which eating habits play a part fall into three main categories: cardiovascular; gastrointestinal; metabolic. They include major killer diseases such as ischaemic heart disease, cerebrovascular disease and cancer; together these are responsible for the death of more than 50% of the British population. Less severe diseases, such as dental caries, are also of major public health importance because of their very high prevalence.

Disease generally results from the combined effect of several causative factors; a bad eating habit is frequently one such factor. Overt disease occurs in those individuals who, because of their genetic make-up, cannot adapt sufficiently to the stresses imposed upon them by their way of life. Individual variation in behaviour and in susceptibility to disease are important factors in modern medicine.

We face a situation, therefore, in which the population has been protected against the ravages of the major killer diseases of infective origin, but instead the public health is put at risk by "self abuse". It is insufficient merely to adopt a therapeutic approach. However good the treatment of disease, prevention is a far more worthwhile aim and diseases of affluent societies are largely preventable. We have to ask, though, whether current medical and educational policies and practices are appropriate and sufficient for such a task.

Be that as it may, in order to deal with the health problems in affluent societies today a first step must be to define the nature and extent of the problem: it is also necessary to define what is known and equally what is not known about the causes of modern diseases. Health, education and other policies and strategies then need to be decided, and both corporate and individual responsibilities identified. In other words, we have to decide what action is necessary and possible and then we have to act, and act decisively.

In this book many aspects of the problem are examined. The nature, prevalence and cost of diseases in which diet plays a part are described. The problems of some special groups, especially the young, are examined in some detail. The case is made for greater surveillance of eating behaviour and health status. Nearly half of the book is devoted to the critical problem of communication—by what means can existing knowledge be used more effectively to promote the health and welfare of the whole community.

The book leads all those in a position of influence to reflect upon their own individual responsibilities in the prevention of disease and the promotion of optimal health. One aspect of the need was expressed at the conference by a health visitor working in the community who asked that more should be done to provide appropriate and readily available in-service training in nutrition. Her sentiments were echoed by those in other professions, including nurses and schoolteachers.

If this text causes the leaders of the professions to re-evaluate the nutrition component in the basic and in-service training of their members, it will have achieved an important function. If it also encourages government to give additional priority to preventive medicine, including nutrition education, a major step forward will have been taken.

June 1981

Michael R. Turner

Acknowledgements

I should like to thank all who contributed to the success of the conference on which this book is based, but especially: Dr R. J. L. Allen, OBE, Dr W. P. T. James, Professor J. McKenzie, Professor I. Macdonald, Professor J. N. Morris, CBE, and Dr R. G. Whitehead who worked with me to produce the scientific programme; Miss Brenda Ewington who undertook the secretarial work relating the scientific programme; and Mr P. M. Victory, OBE MC, Secretary to the BNF, who dealt with administrative matters with the able support of other members of the BNF Staff, Mrs Eleanor Fox, Mrs Valerie Hobbs and Miss Sonia Willie. I should like also to express my gratitude to Dr Gerard Vaughan, Minister of State for Health, who gave the opening address at the conference, to the other contributors, and to the three chairmen: Sir Henry Yellowlees, KCB, Professor Ian Macdonald and Professor John Treasure.

Michael R. Turner

Contents

The Prevalence of Diet-related Diseases in Britain

W. P. T. James, J. Powles and D. R. R. Williams

MRC Dunn Clinical Nutrition Centre,
Addenbrooke's Hospital, Cambridge

There is still a tendency to view nutritional aspects of health solely in terms of the presence or absence of nutritional diseases. This view of nutrition stems from the rapid advances in knowledge on the role of vitamins in metabolism which developed before and after the Second World War. Progress was so rapid at this time and the implications of good nutrition for health so evident that Government used legislative measures to ensure that the population was well fed. Care was taken not only to supplement staple foods, e.g. flour, with minerals and vitamins, but to provide also a cheap infant milk formula (National Dried Milk), free milk for schoolchildren and a carefully controlled school lunch programme.

These measures seemed to be the culmination of a remarkable two decades of nutrition research stemming from the discovery of the vitamin to the wartime experiments of McCance and Widdowson on nutritional aspects of bread. There then seemed few problems of public health importance which warranted attention. The impetus for nutritionists had gone and most of the high quality nutrition research by British research workers was subsequently undertaken overseas, where protein-energy malnutrition was becoming of major concern.

The pendulum is now swinging once more, with increasing interest being taken in nutritional aspects of health in Britain, stimulated by the medical profession's recognition that many of the UK's major public health problems play a crucial role. Unfortunately, the nutritional world has been slow to react to this new challenge, and given the early pre-occupation with the relatively simple task of identifying the importance of a vitamin in a deficiency disease, there has been considerable reluctance to accept that in many of the diseases of affluence there are a number of interacting factors which have to be disentangled before the role of the nutrition components can be identified.

The purpose of this chapter is to summarize some of the available evidence which illustrates these interactions and to show how one needs to take account of evidence from a variety of sources; from epidemiological studies of cohorts being monitored in prospective epidemiological investigations; from clinical work on patients; from detailed physiological studies which display the important interaction of individual susceptibility and diet; and from nutrition studies in animals, particularly non-human primates. Animal studies have often been neglected in nutritional research and any information gained has been dismissed on the grounds that *homo sapiens* is too different from other species for the information gained to be relevant. While this distinction between species is important when dealing with some aspects of metabolism, there are many parallels in the responses of animals and man to diet and true species' differences in metabolism can now be put in perspective. Work on non-human primates is particularly important since their metabolism is very similar to that of man. This work will therefore be included in the assessment of the problem of diet-related diseases.

The prevalence of diseases in Britain

Figure 1 illustrates the changes which have occurred over the last eighty years in the mortality pattern of the British population. The current figures are based on data for 1977 and presuppose that those born in that year will experience the same environmental factors in their lifetime as those operating in 1977. The figure shows that this country has seen a remarkable change in life expectancy. The mortality of children has been practically eliminated as many infectious diseases have been brought under control. This has followed the improvement in the economic, social and nutritional conditions of children and has been helped by the introduction of immunization and anti-microbial drugs. Similar factors have helped to reduce mortality from infections in late adolescence and adult life. However, the fall in adult mortality has been very much less than that predicted from the data on children. Instead of mortality falling to only 8% of that observed at the turn of the century, as in children, the mortality of young and middle aged women has fallen only to 42% and that of men only to 64% of that observed eighty years ago. This reduction in mortality of men and women of working age is apparent throughout Europe, but the improvement in mortality rates has been very uneven and the more affluent countries are not necessarily those showing the greatest improvement. Thus Greek men and women have a substantially lower mortality rate than that

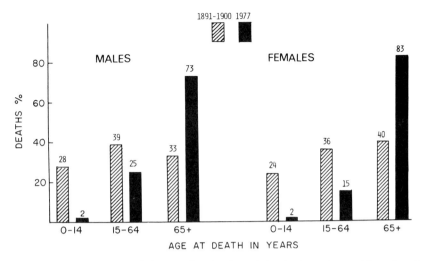

Figure 1   A comparison of the age distribution of deaths in males and females at the beginning of the century and in 1977.

found in Finland or the United Kingdom. England and Wales, however, do have lower death rates than Scotland or Ireland, where only two-thirds of 15-year-old boys may expect to reach retiring age (Table I).

The reason for the poorer response in adult mortality is well known. Deaths from infectious disease have been replaced by deaths from other conditions—the most important in terms of life expectancy are listed in Table II, where data have been recalculated from mortality statistics to display the more important factors contributing to the loss of working years before retirement at the age of 65 years. Death rates do not, of course, give a complete picture of the prevalence of those conditions which lead to high

Table I

Mortality risk before 65 years of 15-year-olds in 1977 (World Health Statistics Annual, 1979).

	Males (%)	Females (%)
Greece (1976)	21	11
Sweden	22	12
England and Wales	26	15
Scotland	31	18
Northern Ireland	31	18
Finland	34	14

medical costs and working years lost before death. This aspect of health economics is considered in the following chapter. Whichever method of expression is used, it is apparent that cardiovascular disease and cancer contribute very substantially to both morbidity and mortality. These conditions, therefore, deserve study to see to what extent environmental factors contribute.

Ischaemic heart disease

Ischaemic heart disease is the major cardiovascular disease responsible for deaths below the age of 65 years, and itself constitutes the single most important cause of deaths in the working men (Table II). It is not surprising, therefore, that such an enormous effort has been made to disentangle the principal factors involved in its aetiology.

Table II

Major causes of death from 15—64 years in England and Wales
(O.P.C.S. Mortality Statistics, 1977).

	Males	Females
Ischaemic heart disease	23	10
Hypertension and other heart diseases	3	5
Cerebrovascular disease	4	6
	30	21
Cancer	22	35
Pneumonia and chronic respiratory diseases	7	7
Injuries (excluding suicide and homicide)	17	9
Other	23	28
	69	79
TOTAL[a]	100	100

[a]Excluding congenital and perinatal causes. Calculations based on years of life lost.

There can be little doubt that the severity and prevalence of ischaemic heart disease are profoundly affected by environmental factors. The marked differences in the severity of ischaemic heart disease in different countries support this concept, although one may be concerned that genetic differences between populations might influence this variation. Indeed, different diagnostic criteria could in part explain the reported differences in the prevalence of heart disease in, for example, rural Africa compared with the United States. There is a large number of studies, however, which resolves this problem. Shaper's series of meticulous investigations in East Africa has shown that ischaemic heart disease is comparatively rare in these communities (Shaper, 1972). Vaughan and Miall (1979) have conducted similar studies in the Gambia and shown remarkably low rates of electro-cardiographic abnormalities in rural Gambians. Blacks in Jamaica and the United States have a much higher rate of ischaemic heart disease. Pathological studies have confirmed the striking differences in coronary atherosclerosis in different communities (McGill, 1968), so difficulty in the diagnosis of this condition is not the explanation for differences in the reported prevalence of heart disease.

Two pieces of evidence can now be used to deal with the problem of genetic differences between populations. The first argument relates to studies on migrants. If migrant groups show an increased incidence of ischaemic heart disease, then this is unlikely to signify the impact of new environmental factors. This is a powerful argument unless one considers migrants to be a genetically selected group representing the more enterprising and intense members of their community who decide to look for greater opportunities in another country. On this basis one might claim that those who migrate may well be temperamentally unstable and therefore more susceptible to heart disease. However, in the Boston – Irish studies, brothers living in the USA and Ireland were found to have such a marked difference in heart disease that genetic selection of migrants is unlikely to explain the low prevalence of heart disease in Ireland (Brown *et al.,* 1970). If one argued that the link between the tendency to migrate and the genetic susceptibility to heart disease was so strong that this selection operated even on brothers, then one would have to argue that Ireland had been substantially depleted over the last hundred years of coronary-prone individuals! This genetic argument cannot be sustained in view of the secular increase in heart disease in Ireland itself over the last twenty to thirty years. Studies of Japanese migrating to different communities add force to the environmental basis of ischaemic heart disease. Japanese who migrated to Hawaii have been found to have an age-adjusted prevalence rate for definite ischaemic heart disease, determined by electrocardiograph, which is no different from the rates in native Japanese. Migrants who went to live in California, however, show more than a two-fold increase in heart disease (Marmot *et al.,* 1975). Thus migration, as such, does not automatically mean that a group will have a higher rate of ischaemic heart disease and there is no evidence that the Californian Japanese are genetically different from the Hawaiian Japanese.

Further support for the environmental case comes from the clear evidence that there has been an increase in the death rates of young men and women

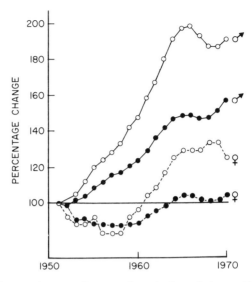

Figure 2   The changes in mortality rates from ischaemic heart disease in England and Wales. Changes for men: 35—44 years O–O ; 45—54 years ●–●. Changes for women: 35—44 years O– –O; 45—54 years ●– –● (DHSS, 1974)

in England and Wales (Fig. 2). The percentage of deaths in 35- to 44-year-old men almost doubled in less than twenty years. The percentage change reflects a true increase in the rate of deaths from heart attacks and is not a reflection of a decline in deaths related to other diseases. Clearly, genetic factors cannot account for this increase in ischaemic heart disease and changing criteria for diagnosis cannot be considered to be the explanation.

The evidence for an environmental effect has been set out in sequence because too often there has been a tendency, even among experts, to dismiss this epidemiological data as either unsound or of too general a nature to be very relevant to the problem of the pathogenesis of ischaemic heart disease. Those scientists who wish to emphasize the albeit important role of genetic susceptibility to heart disease (see below) often neglect the strong epidemiological evidence showing the major changes in the pattern of cardiovascular disease in genetically heterogeneous populations; these changes must reflect the impact of environmental factors.

The pathological process of atherosclerosis

Arterial wall changes and the development of atherosclerosis begin in childhood and adolescence. Originally the fatty streaks of the intimal wall of children were linked with the fully developed atherosclerotic lesion of the adult, but not all types of fatty streak are now considered to be precursors of the intimal proliferation and the lipid deposition characteristic of the adult disease. McGill (1974) has described several types of fatty streak. The first dominant lesion affects the arteries of children from all populations irrespective of the prevalence of atherosclerosis. These lesions increase rapidly in adolescence and occur more commonly in girls and in Negroes: both groups have a lower rate of atherosclerosis than that of white adult males. The lesions also occur irrespective of the socio-economic circumstance of the children, another known factor relating to the prevalence of atherosclerosis. On a pathological basis, the fatty streaks consist of an intracellular collection of lipid which leads to the formation of foam cells, but there is no new connective tissue growth. The epidemiological and pathological evidence, therefore, argues against these streaks being an early lesion of atherosclerosis.

A second type of fatty streak occurs in early adulthood, particularly in atherosclerotic-prone populations. Extracellular lipid accumulates and this may in part follow the disintegration of foam cells, cellular necrosis and cholesterol crystal deposition; connective tissue proliferation is also present so these lesions can then be considered to be the precursors of atherosclerotic plaques.

During childhood the aorta undergoes a series of changes with diffuse intimal thickening accompanied by a marked increase in the concentration of plasma very low density lipoprotein (VLDL) within the arterial wall. Although these changes affect particularly the abdominal aorta, intimal thickening of the coronary arteries also occurs, the degree of thickening correlating with the prevalence of clinical ischaemic heart disease in the adult population (Vlodaver *et al.,* 1969). Whether the steadily increasing blood pressure in affluent populations affects these changes is unknown, although increased sub-intimal thickening is noted in children with clinically overt hypertension (Wilens, 1951). The accumulation of lipid within the intima is progressive throughout childhood with a steady increase in free cholesterol, phospholipid and triglyceride. By the end of adolescence there is a marked and progressive increase in cholesterol ester and this seems to be in equilibrium with the plasma esterified cholesterol, since its fatty acid composition is similar. The similarity in fatty acid pattern of these later arterial changes distinguishes the pathological accumulation of lipid from the initial type of fatty streak of childhood which has a relatively higher proportion of the mono-unsaturated fatty acid, oleic acid, and less of the poly-unsaturated fatty acid, linoleic acid, than that found in plasma. In the childhood type of fatty streak the cholesterol appears to be esterified within the smooth muscle cells of the arterial intima and does not accumulate to the same extent.

Proliferation of smooth muscle cells seems to be an important component of atherogenesis. Proliferation is enhanced by any injury of the endothelium, e.g. that induced by smoking; this denudation then allows platelets both to aggregate at the injured site and to release factors, including a low molecular weight protein, which then induces the smooth muscle cells to proliferate. The muscle cells aggregate in layers parallel to the luminal surface of the intima and constitute a significant element of the plaque; they also seem able to synthesize the extracellular tissue matrix, which is one of the key components of atheromatous plaques.

Two recent studies of paediatric disease for which there are animal models have revealed the importance of platelet aggregation in the generation of atherosclerotic plaques. In the autosomal recessive disease of homocystinuria there is a marked increase in atherosclerosis and children tend to die of thrombo-embolic complications. Baboons with the same condition show patchy loss of endothelium. Increased circulating concentrations of homocystine enhance platelet stickiness and increase the clumping of platelets to the denuded endothelial areas. Atherosclerosis then develops but can be limited by the use of dipyridamole which reduces the platelets' adhesiveness (Harker *et al.,* 1976). The other evidence to show that endothelial damage does not necessarily lead to atherosclerosis comes from a study of pigs with von Willebrand's disease (Fuster *et al.,* 1978). These animals have a similar platelet defect to that found in humans and do not develop the usual arterial lesions when fed high cholesterol diets, despite the diet-induced areas of denuded endothelium on the vessel walls.

**Environmental factors in the development of
ischaemic heart disease**

Numerous studies have shown that in western societies the three most important risk factors for ischaemic heart disease are smoking, high blood pressure and an elevated serum concentration of cholesterol. All three factors show a graded effect. This is illustrated in Fig. 3, which summarizes the evidence from a very large collaborative United States study (Pooling Project Research Group, 1978). Smoking is an important factor in the development of ischaemic heart disease and about half of the excess mortality in smokers in the UK and USA is due to cardiovascular disease. At any level of risk from the other risk factors, i.e. elevated blood pressure or serum cholesterol, cigarette smoking in the environment of both the USA and the UK doubles the risk of a myocardial infarct. In men below 45 years of age smoking increases the risk of ischaemic heart disease ten-fold (Borhani, 1977). The risk is proportional not only to the number of cigarettes smoked, but also to the duration of smoking, being the highest in the group who started smoking before the age of 20 years. The continuing deleterious effect of smoking in adult life is illustrated by the marked decline in the risk of ischaemic heart disease which occurs once a subject stops smoking.

Smoking and its interaction with other environmental factors

Smoking appears to act by damaging the endothelium of the arterioles. This denudation of the endothelium allows the platelets to aggregate on the surface of the vessel and thereby stimulates smooth muscle cells to replicate. These are important features of the atheromatous process, but in experimental animals it is clear that the animals need to be on an atheromatous diet as well as exposed to smoking or carbon monoxide if the arterial lesions are to develop into the clear-cut atherosclerosis found in man.

Parallel epidemiological observations have been made in man. Smoking only seems to lead to progressive atherosclerosis if an appropriate western-style atherogenic diet is fed. Thus despite the widespread habit of smoking and the high prevalence of hypertension in Japan, Japanese men have a low mortality rate from ischaemic heart disease (Worth *et al.*, 1975). This is illustrated in Table III, which shows the greater importance in Japan of strokes (which are closely related to hypertensive disease) but the much lower rate of deaths from ischaemic heart disease compared with Japanese living in San Francisco. The prevalence rate of ischaemic heart disease is, of

Table III

Annual mortality rates for Japanese men living in Japan, Honolulu (Hawaii) and San Francisco (California) (Worth *et al.*, 1975).

Age at death (years)		Annual mortality rate per 1000 men		
		Japan	Honolulu	San Francisco
50−54	Strokes	31·4	0·5	−
	IHD[a]	0·4	1·1	1·3
55−59	Strokes	1·5	0·9	0·5
	IHD	1·4	1·7	4·8
60−64	Strokes	5·4	1·1	2·5
	IHD	2·1	3·9	4·9

[a]Ischaemic heart disease.

Preventive Nutrition and Society

course, much higher than the death rate. If prevalence rates are assessed in relation to cigarette smoking has three Japanese communities (Table IV), it becomes clear that cigarette smoking has only a small effect on ischaemic heart disease in Japan, whereas there is a 55% increase in risk in Japanese Californians who smoke. In the Japanese living in Japan the smaller risk associated with smoking in a community of 45- to 40-year-old men occurs

Table IV

The differential effects of smoking and other environmental factors in Japanese men living in Japan, Hawaii and California.[a]

| | Prevalence of ischaemic heart disease No. per 1000 age adjusted | | |
	Never smoked	Ex-smoker	Current smoker
Japan	14·0	26·0	19·6
Hawaii	20·8	42·9	24·4
California	45·7	62·0	70·7

[a]Prevalence rates based on studies of 1343 men living in Japan, 7980 in Hawaii and 1773 in California. Ischaemic heart disease was diagnosed either on the basis of a Minnesota classification of electrocardiographic abnormalities or from evidence of angina or a myocardial infarct derived from the London School of Hygiene Cardiovascular Questionnaire. Data from Marmot *et al.* (1975). The Japanese group of smokers did not contain as many very heavy smokers as in the California group of smokers so the Japanese— Californian differences in the ratio for current smokers may be exaggerated.

with an average serum cholesterol of 180 mg/100 ml (SEM 2·2) in Californian Japanese of equivalent age (Nichaman *et al.,* 1975). The difference in the prevalence of ischaemic heart disease among the non-smoking groups in the three communities is yet more striking with a three-fold difference in risk between the Japanese and Californian environments. Further evidence for a disparity between the consumption of tobacco and the development of heart disease comes from international comparisons of smoking and heart disease. Table V shows that Greece has the same tobacco consumption rate as the UK, but less than one third of the death rate from ischaemic heart disease. The Japanese data, already discussed, are even more striking. Clearly, therefore, smoking is of great public health significance in our community, especially because of the important interaction with other environmental factors. It is this interaction which we must recognize if we are to make much head-way in understanding the basis of ischaemic heart disease. Smoking, hypertension and a high serum cholesterol are not independent risk factors: the effect of hypertension and of hypercholesterolaemia is less in non-smokers.

Table V

Smoking and ischaemic heart disease (IHD) (O.P.C.S.
Mortality Statistics, 1969—73).

	Mortality rate[a] IHD Men 35—74 years	Tobacco consumption (lb/year)
UK	702	6·2
USA	794	9·2
Japan	115	7·2
Greece	205	6·3

[a]Mortality rate is age averaged per 100,000 for 1973.

Dietary factors in the development of ischaemic heart disease

Keys (1980) and his colleagues in their studies of the risk factors associated with ischaemic heart disease in seven very different communities in widely scattered parts of the world, found a relationship between the level of serum cholesterol in a community and the risk of developing ischaemic heart disease. This association between elevated serum cholesterol and ischaemic heart disease has since been confirmed in cohort studies of men living in different parts of the USA (see Fig. 3). The problem, though, was to demonstrate whether the elevated cholesterol concentration in the blood itself affects the atherosclerotic process or whether the high serum cholesterol is only an index of the individual's metabolism, with another process being involved in the pathophysiological basis of atherosclerosis.

The emphasis on serum cholesterol concentration has led to a great deal of confusion in the field because it has been inferred that the dietary cholesterol must be of key significance. The finding that the atherosclerotic plaque contained cholesterol seemed to emphasize the importance of this component of the diet. There then followed a series of animal experiments which assessed the effects of diets containing high concentrations of cholesterol on the amount of cholesterol deposited in the arteries. Once this dietary cholesterol was shown to increase arterial cholesterol deposition, the American Heart Foundation recommended that dietary intakes of cholesterol should be limited in order to reduce serum cholesterol concentrations and reduce the risk of heart disease. It is now clear that saturated fatty acid intake is more important than dietary cholesterol in determining serum cholesterol concentrations.

Keys and his colleagues first showed that the rate of ischaemic heart

Preventive Nutrition and Society

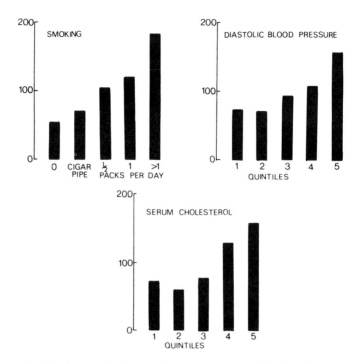

Figure 3   Risk factors for first major coronary event (Pooling Project, 1978).

disease in different communities was proportional to the amount of dietary energy invested in the form of saturated fatty acids. The studies of Japanese migrants also revealed that the lower serum concentration of the Hawaiian and native Japanese was associated with a low intake of total fat, of saturated fatty acids and of dietary cholesterol (Kato *et al.*, 1973). In metabolic studies Keys observed that young men fed a constant fat intake markedly increased their serum cholesterol concentrations when a diet rich in saturated fatty acids was substituted for one rich in polyunsaturated fatty acids (Fig. 4).

The influence of the cholesterol and fatty acid content of the diet on serum cholesterol has been calculated by several investigations from a large number of metabolic studies. Hegsted *et al.* (1965) produced an equation relating changes in diet to changes in serum cholesterol:

$$\Delta Y = 2 \cdot 16 \quad \Delta S - 1 \cdot 65 \quad \Delta P + 6 \cdot 77C - 0 \cdot 53,$$

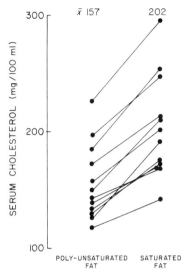

Figure 4   The effect of a saturated fat intake on serum cholesterol. Data from metabolic studies on normal young men (Keys *et al.,* 1959).

where ΔY =   the change in mg/100 ml in serum cholesterol,
S = the amount of saturated triglyceride, expressed as a percentage of dietary energy,
P = the amount of polyunsaturated triglyceride, expressed as a percentage of dietary energy
C = the cholesterol intake in decigrams (not milligrams) per day.

The effect of dietary cholesterol, which is independent of fatty acid intake, is not nearly as great as that of saturated fatty acids. Mono-unsaturated fatty acids are found to be without effect on serum cholesterol.

The unimportance of dietary cholesterol can be appreciated if it is recognized that the change in serum cholesterol concentration equivalent to that displayed in Fig. 4 could be achieved only by completely eliminating the cholesterol from the diet. To halve the intake of cholesterol to about 350 mg/day would involve major changes in diet and this would achieve a reduction in serum cholesterol equal to half the increment observed with saturated fatty acids in Fig. 4. The relatively poor response in serum cholesterol to alterations in dietary cholesterol intake stems from the fact that in man, unlike many experimental animals, the *majority* of the body's supply of cholesterol is synthesized endogenously and not derived from the diet. The cholesterol feeding experiments have proved to be inappropriate models in many cases because, unlike man, many of the species studied showed a marked effect of dietary cholesterol on circulating cholesterol concentration—this difference depending both on the higher absorption rates in the animal models and on a failure to switch off endogenous cholesterol production.

In the experimental animal studies huge increase in cholesterol in the blood vessels were found when dietary cholesterol was increased. It is now recognized that the abnormalities induced in the arteries depended on the dominating influence of dietary cholesterol on serum cholesterol and the abnormality reflected only intense deposition of cholesterol without the development of a typical atherosclerotic lesion. This histological dissociation between cholesterol deposition and atherosclerosis applied to studies on both rodents and non-human primates. Thus, in due course, cholesterol feeding experiments may well be seen as a confusing phase in research on atherosclerosis.

We may ultimately link with this confusion the prominence given at present to the role of "poly-unsaturated" fatty acids in the diet. Figure 4 displays the lower serum cholesterol concentration when a diet rich in poly-unsaturated fatty acids is substituted for a diet high in saturated fatty acids. The lower serum cholesterol concentration reflects both the absence of the saturated fatty acids which promote endogenous synthesis and, as suggested by Hegsted's formula, the specific cholesterol lowering effects of poly-unsaturated fatty acids. This effect of poly-unsaturated fatty acids on cholesterol metabolism does not necessarily link with a specific effect on the atherosclerotic process and it should not be assumed that manipulating the concentration of the well-established risk factor, serum cholesterol, will necessarily reduce the development of atherosclerosis. Reducing serum cholesterol by artificial means, e.g. by the use of the drug clofibrate, does reduce the incidence of heart attacks (Committee of Principal Investigators, 1978) but the effect is not striking and unfortunately is marred by the greater risk of other complications (Committee of Principal Investigators, 1980).

The importance of specific types of fatty acids in the atherosclerotic process

Assessing the relative importance of different types of fatty acid in the development of atherosclerois is difficult and time-consuming even when studies are conducted in animals. Several experiments on non-human primates have now clearly shown that certain types of dietary fat can lead to progressive atherosclerosis of a type which simulates that found in man. The addition to the diet of substantial amounts of peanut oil, for example, leads to progressive atherosclerosis. The severity of this condition on peanut oil feeding far exceeds that predicted simply from the ratio of saturated to poly-unsaturated fatty acids and may relate to the high concentration of unusual long-chain saturated fatty acids (Vesselinovitch *et al.*, 1980). Primate studies which assess the relative importance of individual fatty acids are not available, nor, surprisingly, are there carefully controlled studies to assess the protective effect of adding poly-unsaturated fatty acids to an atherogenic diet rather than substituting one completely for the other. Studies by Renaud and his colleagues on rodents, however, suggest that some saturated fatty acids, e.g. C_{14} myristic acid and the longer-chain behenic and arachidic acids may have particularly severe adverse effects on platelet function. There is also increasing evidence from metabolic epidemiology that changes in fatty acid consumption affect platelet function and relate to the dietary patterns and prevalence rate of atherosclerosis in different communities (Renaud *et al.*, 1979).

Further impetus for a reassessment of the role of specific fatty acids has come from the work of Dyerberg and his colleagues. They noted that Eskimos leading their traditional lives consumed a high-fat diet, but did not appear to suffer from ischaemic heart disease until they transferred to a western diet which contained a smaller fat content. Dyerberg noted that the type of fat eaten by Eskimos was derived principally from seals and was very different from that found in many animals. The diet contained much higher quantities of the long-chain poly-unsaturated fatty acids derived indirectly from those synthesized by the plankton on which the seals feed. It was suggested that eicosapentaenoic acid, i.e. $C_{20} : 5\Omega - 3$, was deficient in many western diets and that this unusual fatty acid affected prostaglandin and thromboxane synthesis and platelet function in a manner quite different from that normally induced by arachidonic acid, the derivative of the essential fatty acid linoleic acid. This theory emphasizes our limited knowledge of the way in which specific fatty acids and their derivatives might work (Dyerberg *et al.*, 1978).

On this basis it is quite possible that a markedly different view of the key dietary factors involved in the development of ischaemic heart disease will emerge in the next few years. Nevertheless, on the basis of current ideas it seems reasonable to consider the primate experiments, human metabolic and epidemiological work as consistent with the concept that some factor in the dietary fats consumed by western societies is responsible for ischaemic heart disease. Primate studies increasingly suggest that the atherosclerotic process can be reversed (Malinow, 1980), but this is a very slow process. Given the difficulty encountered in resolving atheromatous plaques filled with fibrous material and lipid, it is not surprising that studies on the effects of dietary changes in patients who have suffered a heart attack often fail to show an improvement in the subsequent mortality. With our incomplete knowledge of fatty acid metabolism and its relationship to atheroma, it may also seem not too surprising that primary prevention trials based on the use of diets enriched with poly-unsaturated fatty acids have had only a small effect on the subsequent frequency of heart attacks.

Genetics and ischaemic heart disease

Although the evidence available supports the key role of diet in the development of atherosclerosis, there is an importa.lt genetic component which is often misunderstood.

Figure 4, in addition to showing the effects of saturated fatty acids on serum cholesterol concentrations, also illustrates the remarkable range in serum cholesterol to be found in normal young men fed the same diet. The two-fold range in serum cholesterol on the basal diet is exaggerated by feeding saturated fatty acids and those with the higher basal serum cholesterol concentrations show the greatest response. On this basis it is evident why there has often been difficulty in establishing a simple relationship in individuals between the saturated fatty acid intake and their serum cholesterol; the serum level is the result of the interaction between the saturated fatty acid intake and the individual's susceptibility.

This is illustrated in Fig. 5, which shows that for each community in Keys' seven-country study there is no relationship between saturated fatty acid intake and the serum cholesterol values. Again we see the 2- to 3-fold range in cholesterol values which could be predicted from the metabolic studies depicted in Fig. 4. Yet, when the range of saturated fatty acid intake is expanded sufficiently by the inclusion of several communities, the relationhip between fatty acid intake and serum cholesterol then becomes apparent. In theory it could be argued that the variable response does not reflect an innate, genetically determined programming of cholesterol metabolism but the effect of some environmental factor operating in early life and thereby programming the individual's subsequent metabolic response. Nevertheless, it seems most likely that the variable responsiveness reflects some of the effects of polygenic inheritance and that this, at least in part, explains the similarity of children's and parents' serum cholesterol; differences in household fat intakes are unlikely to vary enough to explain the marked differences in the serum cholesterol levels of different households.

Sometimes the relationship between diet and serum cholesterol does seem

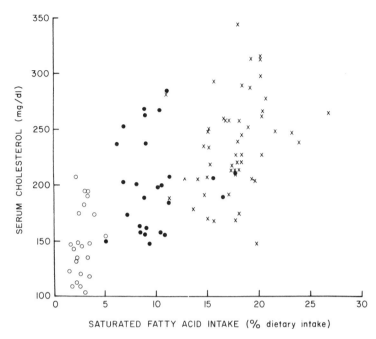

Figure 5   The relationship between the saturated fatty acid intake and the serum cholesterol concentration in three communities: Tanushimaru ○ ; Crete ● ; Zutphen × (Keys and Kimura, 1970).

apparent even within a single population. Thus in a study of six-month-old infants, 6% of whom had serum cholesterol levels above 200 mg/100 ml, there was greater energy, protein and milk consumption in the hyper-cholesterolaemic group (Vobecky *et al.,* 1979). A strong correlation was also found between the poly-unsaturated/saturated fatty acid ratio of the diet and serum total cholesterol levels in 6- to 10-month-old children (Anderson *et al.,* 1979). However, in schoolchildren no such relationship was found. Apart from differences in individual responsiveness, there may also have been a greater variability in life style and in the intake of other nutrients, e.g. sugar and dietary fibre (Van der Haar and Kromhout, 1978; Weidman *et al.,* 1978) in these older children.

Many surveys have shown that there is a familial aggregation of heart disease although estimates of risk vary depending to some extent on the method used to assess it. Rose (1964) found a 3-fold excess mortality from ischaemic heart disease in relatives of male survivors of a myocardial infarct. In a more detailed analysis, Slack (1975) found that there is a 3- to 7-fold increase in risk of heart disease at a comparatively young age if a first degree relative has a myocardial infarct. These data can be used to predict risk in children since they indicate that a boy's risk of developing ischaemic heart disease before the age of 55 years will be increased at least 5-fold if his father is already affected, whereas a daughter has approximately half this risk. However, the application of these risk factors is limited since parents tend to have their children well before they themselves develop overt disease. Attempts have therefore been made to establish whether measurements of serum lipids can indicate risk of ischaemic heart disease in children.

Several of the unusual conditions of familial hyperlipidaemia can be diagnosed in childhood, and these are associated with abnormalities of lipid metabolism which reflect discrete, genetically inherited diseases. Children with the homozygous form of familial hypercholesterolaemia are prone to develop ischaemic heart disease in the second decade of life. The heterozygous form accounts, in part, for the familial aggregation of coronary artery disease in the population as it affects approximately 1 in 500 individuals, and can also be diagnosed in childhood by measuring the serum cholesterol. The risk of a child having heterozygous hypercholestero-laemia is 1 in 2 if a parent is a known case and the genetic risk of a child being affected is 1 in 8 if the parent has suffered an early myocardial infarct (Paterson and Slack, 1972). Testing a child in these circumstances is well worthwhile in coronary-prone families and if a parent is known to be heterozygous. Half the boys and 12% of girls with the heterozygous form of hypercholesterolaemia will have their first heart attack by the age of 50 years (Slack, 1969). Diagnosis is made either by finding an increased concentration of β-lipoprotein cholesterol in umbilical cord blood (Kwiterovich *et al.,* 1973), or by finding a total serum cholesterol concentration above 264 mg/100 ml (6·8 mmol/1) at the age of 1 year.

Children with a serum cholesterol which exceeds the 95th percentile on two occasions have first and second degree relatives with much higher serum cholesterol concentrations than those of children with a normal or low serum cholesterol. There is also about a 4-fold increase in the number of deaths from ischaemic heart disease in relatives of children with a persistently high serum cholesterol (Lauer *et al.,* 1977).

Although serum cholesterol is a crude predictor of the risk of ischaemic heart disease, there is no direct evidence as yet that children with serum cholesterol concentrations in the upper percentile range are more prone to ischaemic heart disease in later life. However, it is known that children found to have an elevated serum cholesterol tend to remain with high values so that there is a rank correlation of serum cholesterol over a four-year period of 0·61 (Clarke *et al.,* 1976). A child's serum cholesterol at the age of 4−9 years tends to resemble that of his or her parents as well as of siblings and the correlation is greater than the recognized parent-child associations for blood pressure (Johnson *et al.,* 1965). This could either mean that children share the same environmental influences which determine serum cholesterol or, more probably that their common genetic make-up influences the response in cholesterol metabolism to dietary factors.

More refined indices of risk for ischaemic heart disease are now being found. A *low* concentration of cholesterol in the high density lipoprotein (HDL) fraction of the blood has now been found to be a better predictor of ischaemic heart disease than either an elevated concentration of total cholesterol or of the concentrations in the very low density lipoprotein fraction (Miller *et al.,* 1977). Conversely, congenital abnormalities of lipoprotein metabolism where high density lipoprotein cholesterol levels are high as in hyper-alpha-lipoproteinaemia or hypo-beta-lipoproteinaemia are associated with longevity and a reduced incidence of myocardial infarction in first degree relatives (Glueck *et al.,* 1976, 1977). Several further epidemiological studies have now shown an inverse relationship between the traditional risk factor for ischaemic heart disease—an elevated VLDL cholesterol—and the more specific risk factor, a low HDL cholesterol concentration. Nupuf and Sutherland (1979) have also observed recently that adolescent children of fathers who have ischaemic heart disease before the age of 55 years have lower concentrations of HDL cholesterol than children of unaffected men; this difference is independent of fasting triglyceride concentrations, cigarette smoking, obesity, diet and physical activity, all of which are known to affect HDL cholesterol concentrations. These HDL levels have also been shown to be similar in Dutch schoolchildren from the same family (Haar and Krombout, 1978). In the general population there is a strong resemblance between the HDL cholesterol of the child and those of his parents. Clearly both genetic and environmental factors contribute to these strong associations in blood lipids.

We may conclude that individual susceptibility to dietary factors makes a substantial difference to the chances of an individual's having a myocardial infarction but, when considering the problem of ischaemic heart disease in the population of the United Kingdom, we must recognize the important interactions of risk factors as illustrated in Fig. 6. For the Japanese community on a traditional diet the dietary circle barely overlaps the others so that, despite individual risks and the high prevalence of cigarette smoking and hypertension, this society has surprisingly little ischaemic heart disease.

Table VI summarizes the differences in rate of coronary artery disease in Europe and the secular changes in mortality—the data is taken from Byington and his colleagues' recent analyses of statistics on coronary artery disease in different countries (Byington *et al.,* 1979). Clearly there are major differences in the risk of coronary artery disease in the different countries of

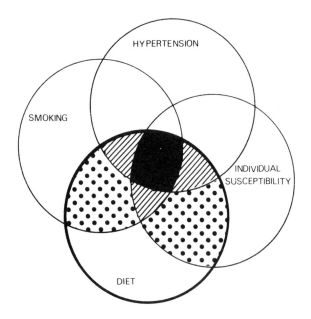

Figure 6 A scheme to display the interactions of smoking, diet, high blood pressure and individual susceptibility in determining the incidence of myocardial infarction.

Table VI

Age-averaged mortality rates[a] from ischaemic heart disease in different countries and the changes calculated from 1969 to 1975. (From corrected Tables 23 and 24, page 373, of Byington et al., 1979.)

Country	Men aged 35−74			Women aged 35−74		
	1969	1975	% change	1969	1975	% change
Belgium	445	429	−3·7	171	155	−9·4
Netherlands	479	495	+3·4	171	160	−6·5
UK	679	697	+2·6	248	248	0
Ireland	658	698	+6·1	288	287	−0·1
France	195	211[b]	+8·2	71	71[b]	0
Germany	427	468	+9·5	141	156	+10·8
Italy	307	300[b]	−2·3	132	119[b]	−9·8
Denmark	566	589	+4·0	236	213	−9·7
USA	865	717	−17·1	359	282	−21·4

[a]Rates are averaged from the rates for the four 10-year age groups 35−44, 45−54, 55−64 and 65−74.
[b]Change calculated from 1969 to 1974.

the European Economic Community and there is very little evidence of any improvement in recent years, except in Belgium and Italy.

An analysis of the major risk factors for ischaemic heart disease viz. elevated serum cholesterol, increased blood pressure and cigarette smoking suggests that in American men 63% of all cases of ischaemic artery disease before the age of 65 years are attributable to less favourable levels of these three risk factors (Byington *et al.,* 1979). Estimates of the relative contribution of each of these three risk factors to ischaemic heart disease mortality can be extracted from the data given for an 8·6-year follow-up of men aged 50 at entry to the Pooling Project (1978). Table VII shows that small changes in the average blood pressure of the population could account for 30% of the fall in total mortality and 20% of the fall in mortality from ischaemic heart disease observed in American whites between 1950 and 1970. Substantial changes in serum cholesterol as such would be needed to produce marked falls in mortality. This does not, of course, mean that this is the extent to which dietary factors as such could affect mortality rates.

Table VII

Contributions of change in individual major risk factors to expected decrease in ischaemic heart disease (IHD) and mortality from all causes (Byington *et al.,* 1979).

Variable	Change in risk factor	Change in IHD mortality %	Change in total mortality %
Serum cholesterol, mean (mg/dl)	235−210	−4·4 (40)[a]	−1·2 (7)
Diastolic blood pressure, mean (mmHg)	86·0−84·3	−2·2 (20)	−4·9 (30)
Cigarette smoking (%)	55−40	−4·5 (41)	−10·5 (63)

[a] % of total fall in mortality accounted for by change in particular risk factor.

Hypertension

High blood pressure is not normally considered to be a diet-related disease. Yet we know that environmental influences must exert a role of key importance since hypertension is considered to be one of the most prevalent of the major diseases in our society and the whole group of cardiovascular diseases are the main cause of death in middle-aged people, especially men, in most industrialized countries. Although ischaemic heart disease is the commonest manifestation of cardiovascular disease in Europe, hypertension markedly increases the risk of ischaemic heart disease, particularly in those societies where obesity (Alexander *et al.*, 1975) hyper-cholesterolaemia and smoking (Borhani, 1977) are prevalent.

The prevalence of hypertension in a country is closely related to the death rate from cerebrovascular disease and there are well substantiated secular trends which add substance to the view that the degenerative changes of the cerebral vessels are linked pathologically to hypertension (Joosens, 1973). In Britain the prevalence of hypertension in adults is about 15%. This figure is similar to that found in 47- to 54-year-old males in Göteborg, Sweden, with systolic blood pressures over 175 mmHg (Berglund *et al.*, 1975) and a 15% prevalence in 20- to 40-year-old men in Heidelberg, with blood pressures in excess of 160/95 mmHg. Detailed knowledge of the prevalence of hypertension in different parts of Britain and other EEC countries is not available, despite widespread interest in this topic.

The importance of even mild hypertension in the development of ischaemic heart disease has been reaffirmed by the recently published study on the Hypertension Detection and Follow-up Program (HDFP) (1979), where borderline hypertensives, defined as having a blood pressure between 140/190 and 160/95 mmHg were found to have 20% lower mortality if they were treated with hypotensive drugs. This reduction in death rates affected particularly black men, who are prone both to hypertension and excess

Table VIII

Mortality from all causes in the Heart Detection and Follow-up programme (1979) trial.

Race, sex or age (years)	Deaths % sample S.C.[a]	R.C.[b]	Per cent reduction in mortality for stepped care group
Black men	10·6 (0·9)	13·0 (1·0)	18·5
Black women	5·2 (0·6)	7·2 (0·7)	27·8
White men	5·8 (0·5)	6·8 (0·6)	14·7
White women	4·9 (0·6)	4·8 (0·6)	−2·1
30−49	3·3 (0·4)	3·5 (0·4)	5·7
50−59	6·2 (0·7)	8·3 (0·6)	25·3
60−69	12·7 (1·0)	15·2 (1·0)	16·4

[a]S.C. (stepped care) group received detailed specific treatment.
[b]R.C. (referred care) group were simply referred for assessment and treatment to their personal physicians.

morbidity. Table VIII summarizes the effectiveness of a reduction in blood pressure on death rates.

The HDFP study analysis to show whether the reduction in mortality of both borderline hypertensives and those with definite hypertension (i.e. with a blood pressure above 160/95 mmHg), resulted from a reduction in the number of people who developed myocardial infarction is still awaited. However, analyses based on single-cause coding of death certificates showed not only a 45% reduction in cardiovascular disease, but 26% fewer deaths attributable to myocardial infarction. In the previous Veterans Administration Study (1967, 1970) the reduced mortality was accounted for by a reduced rate of stroke and congestive heart failure; the reduction in the rate of myocardial infarction failed to achieve statistical significance. The progressively increased risk of myocardial infarction with increasing degrees of hypertension (see Fig. 3) strongly suggests that the prevention of hypertension would contribute substantially to the lowering of the rate of myocardial infarction within a community.

Joossens (1980) has recently analysed the changing rate of cardiovascular disease in several European countries. Table IX shows that there has been an appreciable decline in cerebrovascular mortality in several countries,

Table IX

Mortality trends in the EEC since 1968.[a] Age adjusted 45—64 years; significant % change calculated for 10 years.

Country	Analysis from 1968 until	Cerebrovascular mortality		Coronary mortality	
		Male	Female	Male	Female
Belgium	1977	− 33·6	− 34·2	− 16·5	− 24·9
The Netherlands	1977	− 11·5	− 30·2	—	—
England and Wales	1977	− 25·0	− 26·4	+ 6·8	+ 13·9
Scotland	1976	—	− 13·4	—	+ 14·8
Northern Ireland	1975	—	—	+ 24·9	—
Ireland	1975	—	− 30·9		
France	1974	− 18·4	− 22·1	+ 24·3	—
Germany	1975	− 23·0	− 26·3	+ 18·8	+ 15·4
Italy	1974	− 14·3	− 23·3	+ 12·7	—
Denmark	1976	—	—	—	+ 17·8
Luxemburg	1974	+ 70·3	—	+ 20·5	

[a]From Joosens (1980) with the % calculated as

$$\frac{1000 \times \text{yearly slope of the mortality regression line}}{\text{mean mortality over the interval studied}}$$

Only significant changes are shown. Note that the calculations differ from those used to derive data given in Table VI.

little change in others and a marked statistically significant increase in Luxemburg. Coronary artery mortality, however, has shown little decline or even an increase. If the decline in cerebrovascular mortality relates to a reduction in the problem of hypertension, then on this basis one would expect a decline not an increase in coronary mortality. This in turn suggests either that there are reasons other than hypertension for the decline in cerebrovascular mortality, e.g. an improved vitamin C status (Fig. 7), or that the other factors interacting with hypertension to produce ischaemic heart disease are increasing risk factors within the EEC community. These changes in disease pattern in Europe are in marked contrast to the United States, where there has been not only a marked decline in deaths from cerebrovascular disease, but a 20–30% fall in deaths from ischaemic heart disease (Havlik and Feinlab, 1979).

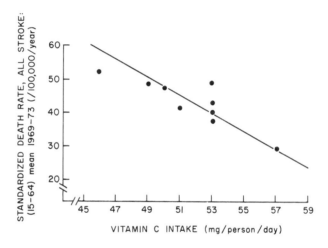

Figure 7   The relationship between the standardized death rate from all strokes in 15- to 64-year-olds and the estimated vitamin C intake in the different regions of England, Wales and Scotland. Dietary data calculated from the National Food Survey (Acheson and Williams, 1979).

Environmental factors and hypertension

The prevalence of hypertension varies throughout the world; in several primitive communities hypertension does not exist and in the Yanomamo Indians the average blood pressure of the population does not increase with age (Fig. 8). In contrast, in Britain and in all other western countries studied, there has been a progressive increase in the average blood pressure

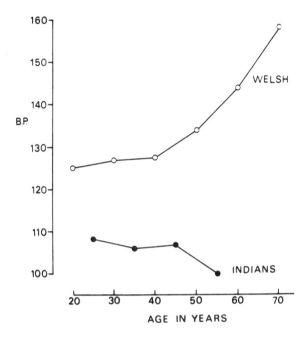

Figure 8 Systolic blood pressure in Welshman and Yanomamo Indians.

in both men and women. This has often been considered to be a natural consequence of ageing. Several studies show that the differences between populations are not the result of genetic differences. Lowenstein (1961) observed two neighbouring Amazonian tribes, the Mundurucus and the Carajas, and monitored their blood pressures. The Mundurucus, who had changed their diet and smoking habits to a western pattern, showed a progressive rise with age in both systolic and diastolic pressure. The Carajas, on the other hand, had not modified their life-style, and had their highest values of blood pressure in young adulthood.

Studies on alterations in the blood pressure of individuals who change their environment reinforce the idea that environmental factors contribute to the prevalence of hypertension. Thus the blood pressures of United States' citizens living in China are lower than those (taken by different observers) in the same individuals living in the USA (Foster, 1927; Tung, 1927; Foster, 1930). Although the authors claimed that the individual's dietary habits had not changed and that the fall in blood pressure related to the reduced pace of life in China, no objective measurements of dietary intake were made.

In East Africa, Samburu tribesmen, when recruited to serve in the British

Army, adopt a British type of diet, increase their weight and have a rise in blood pressure within 12 months. The blood pressure changes are significantly different when compared with age-matched warriors of the same tribe living their traditional lives (Shaper *et al.*, 1969); this cannot be accounted for by the increase in weight.

The problem then becomes one of establishing which environmental factors are responsible for the changes in blood pressure within a population. Few links have been well established, but one of the main factors which has received a great deal of attention is that of sodium intake.

Sodium intake

It has been suggested for several decades that sodium intake is the key to the development of hypertension. A summary of the evidence will be presented here. Figure 9 shows a relationship between the systolic and diastolic blood pressures of different populations and their estimated salt intakes. Dietary assessments have often been far from rigorous and measurement of urinary electrolyte values are only available for eleven of the population groups.

Williams (1980) has identified only two population studies where there appear to be discrepancies between the intake of salt and the prevalence of hypertension. These two studies, by Whyte (1958) and Malhotra (1970), are widely quoted as refuting the hypothesis that sodium intake is related to hypertension. Whyte compared a group of subjects living in the Central Highlands of New Guinea with a group from the Coastal Region; there had been contact between the Coastal group and Europeans over a long period. Mean blood pressures in the younger natives of both groups did not differ significantly from those considered normal for European populations, but blood pressures did not rise with subsequent age in either of the native groups. The mean blood pressures for coastal natives were not greater than those for the highland natives—in fact, mean diastolic pressures were slightly but significantly higher in the latter. The assessment of dietary intake in the highland group was performed by Venkatachalam (quoted by Whyte as a personal communication). Details of this survey have not appeared in the literature and no assessment of the validity of the data can therefore be made. The diet of the coastal natives was assessed by an Australian Government Survey (Hipsley and Clements, 1947) but this makes no *quantitative* reference to the sodium intake. Daily sodium excretion was measured on a small sample of highlanders (20 subjects; mean 30 mEq/24 h) and the coastal natives were "assumed to have a greater (salt) intake" than the highlanders (Whyte, 1958).

Malhotra (1970) compared railway employees living in North and South

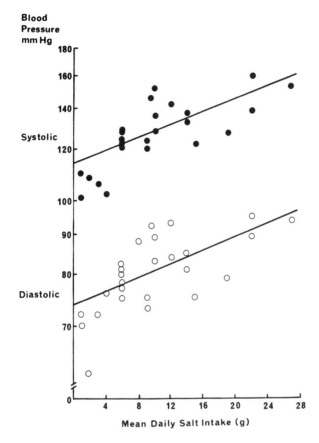

Figure 9 The relationship between blood pressure and estimated salt intakes in males. Redrawn from data of Gleibemann (1973).

India (Delhi and Madras), measuring their blood pressure, serum cholesterol and faecal urobilinogen. Mean blood pressures, by age, were higher in the south than in the north—though not when ponderal index (weight/height²) was taken into account; southerners are more frequently obese than northerners. The prevalence of hypertension in the south was more than double that in the north. This study is often taken as proof that salt intake is unrelated to hypertension, since northern Indians are stated to consume 12–15 g of salt/day compared with 8 g/day for the more hypertension-prone southern Indians. Unfortunately, the dietary data do not refer to the same subjects as those whose blood pressures were measured and relate to 28 pairs of healthy employees who were involved in another study. Estimates of the diet of the Delhi group were made from a sample of the inhabitants of Udaipur, another northern city. Thus the two main studies used epidemiologically to disprove the salt-hypertension hypothesis are inadequate as tests of this relationship.

Where studies have been undertaken of individuals changing their life-style, the relationship of blood pressure to salt intake is maintained. Thus the Samburu tribesmen, on joining the army, increase their salt intake from 3·5 g sodium per day (mainly from meat and milk) to 16 g/day (Shaper *et al.*, 1969), and show a rise in blood pressure. Subjects of similar genetic origin but maintained on lower salt intakes show no such rise. This rise is unlikely to be the result of weight gain since relatively recent recruits, who differ most from their fellow tribesmen in body weight, show less of a difference in blood pressure than longer serving soldiers, whose body weight was lower. The effect of age was taken into account. Japanese living in Japan consume the highest intakes of salt ever recorded (Sasaki, 1964) amounting to between 14 and 22 g/day obtained from salted fish and meats, soy sauce and miso paste. Intakes of salt show variation by prefecture and are positively correlated with prefectural death rates from hypertensive disease (Sasaki, 1962) and from strokes (Takahashi, 1978), the correlation with salt intake being higher than that for fat (Sasaki, 1962).

Evidence on the relationship between salt intake and hypertension within populations

A few studies have shown a relationship between salt intake and hypertension within a country. In Belgium, Joosens *et al.* (1970) found a highly significant relationship between salt intake and systolic blood pressure in men. Several studies, however, fail to find such a relationship. Many of these studies have relied simply on a subjective assessment of salt use by the individuals. Since much less than half the intake of salt comes from salt added to food in cooking or at the table, this approach to salt intake is only qualitative and relates to only some of the salt ingested.

Genetic differences in sodium sensitivity

Dahl (1961) has commented that variation in individual susceptibility to sodium intake is likely. Therefore a relationship in susceptible subjects will be obscured if the evidence from a whole population is considered together. Hypertension is recognized to be a familial condition and a genetic susceptibility is therefore possible.

Dahl (1972) demonstrated that rats could be selectively bred so that one group, when exposed to a high salt diet, displayed extreme hypertension with early deaths from cerebrovascular disease, whereas the other group of rats was salt-resistant and did not develop hypertension with all its complications. The sensitivity to salt could be transferred by renal cross transplantation (Bianchi *et al.*, 1974; Dahl *et al.*, 1974). The salt sensitive rats, before they developed hypertension, characteristically displayed a marked blood response to single doses of sodium: they had an increased, not a decreased, rate of urinary sodium excretion. These animals also displayed abnormalities in sodium transmembrane exchange. Some of these changes preceded the development of hypertension and were also found in animal strains in which hypertension develops spontaneously.

Parallel findings are now becoming apparent in man. Thus Wiggins *et al.* (1978) have found a similar enhanced response to dietary sodium in young normotensive sons of a hypertensive parent. Garay and Meyer (1979) have also found in many normotensive offspring of hypertensive parents and in essential hypertensives (but not in patients with renal hypertension) an erythrocyte defect in the handling of sodium, with an accumulation of intracellular sodium even in the presence of high external potassium ion concentrations.

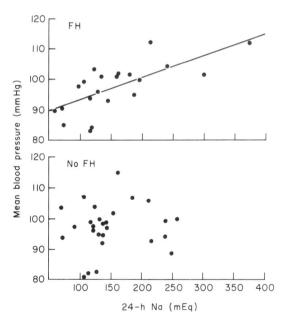

Figure 10 Mean blood pressure and salt intake. Data presented by Pietinen *et al.* (1979) for young adults whose sodium excretion was measured on three sequential days. Those with a family history of hypertension (FH) were found to have a relationship whereas those without a family history (No FH) did not.

These biochemical and physiological tests have recently been accompanied by the demonstration in epidemiological studies that a relationship between sodium intake and blood pressure can be identified provided one selects the susceptible individuals for showing such a relationship and provided the methods for assessing the "usual" blood pressure and salt intake are adequate. Blood pressure does vary from day to day and the first measurement of blood pressure tends to give a high value perhaps because of the anxiety induced by monitoring blood pressure. Similarly salt intake varies from day to day and a single value for sodium excretion fails to take account of this variability. In detailed analyses of this problem Liu *et al.* (1979) have shown that up to nine consecutive measurements of 24-h urine sodium output may be necessary to take account of this daily variability. Pietinen *et al.* (1979) have gone some way towards coping with this problem by monitoring blood pressure and 24-hour urinary sodium outputs for three consecutive days. When this is done it becomes clear that normotensive young adults with hypertensive parents do show a significant relationship between sodium output (an excellent measure of sodium intake) and blood pressure (Fig. 10). Relatives of non-hypertensive subjects do not show this relationship.

The familial aggregation of hypertension

Hypertension runs in families but the problem is one of establishing whether this reflects a shared environment or a common genetic heritage (Miall *et al.*, 1967). An analysis of the blood pressure of first degree relatives shows that their blood pressures resemble each other more than that of spouses, even when the spouses have lived together for more than 10 years. Adults whose blood pressure is more than 1 standard deviation above the mean, i.e. the 16% of the population with the highest blood pressure, have 24% first degree relatives with a similar finding. On the other hand, 16% of the population with the lowest blood pressures have only 2% of first degree relatives with high blood pressure (Miall *et al.*, 1967). A group of asymptomatic children with blood pressures above the 90th percentile for their age had three times as many parents with hypertension as a group of children with blood pressures within the more normal range. Thus it is likely that children display in their centile ranking their genetic susceptibility to hypertension (Londe *et al.*, 1971). Any similarity in the blood pressure of spouses has been ascribed to the tendency for adults to marry individuals of similar age and adiposity, both of which affect blood pressure. These factors seem more important than a shared environment in determining the concordance of their blood pressures. Nevertheless, between 55 and 77% of the variance in systolic blood pressure and between 70 and 87% of the diastolic variance is left to be explained by environmental factors (Miall and Oldham, 1963). It must also be recognized that the polygenic inheritance which seems to characterize the heritability of blood pressure may principally involve the genetic susceptibility to an environmental factor such as sodium rather than an independent genetic programming of arterial changes and blood pressure. The environmental influence may indeed be greater than that observed in a single community, since very marked differences in blood pressure are found in genetically similar races living under different environmental conditions.

Other environmental factors

Body weight

An influence of body weight on blood pressure is well documented. The study of Pacific Islanders by Prior *et al.* (1968), corrected for this influence by regression analysis, showed that the corrected age-specific mean blood pressure estimates differed only by 2–3 mmHg from the means of the values as measured. Thus differences in body weight between the populations were considered unlikely to be the major determinants of the differences in blood pressure.

A similar conclusion was drawn by Shaper *et al.* (1969) from their study of the Samburu soldiers. Recent recruits, who differed most from their tribal controls in terms of their body and mass index, did not show differences in blood pressure, whereas the longer serving soldiers who were no more obese than controls showed considerable increases in blood pressure.

Fat

A direct influence of dietary fat on blood pressure in man has not been established. There is a suggestion that an experimental increase in the $P : S$ ratio of fatty acids can decrease blood pressure in humans (Iacono *et al.*, 1975), though the effect noted might have been the result of decreasing total fat intake. There is no convincing mechanism for an influence of dietary fatty acids on blood pressure, though it has been suggested (Iacono *et al.*, 1975) that changes in prostaglandin synthesis and turnover might provide a mechanism for changes in blood pressure. Rabbits fed fat-enriched diets, showed an increase in arterial blood pressure especially when the fat was of animal origin (Bursty and Firth, 1975). Individual rabbits differed in the magnitude of this response which seems to be independent of weight gain.

The epidemiological evidence on fat is conflicting. Death rates from hypertensive diseases in Japan prefectures are positively correlated with total fat intakes (Sasaki, 1962) as are death rates from the same diseases and from stroke in Standard Regions of Britain (Acheson and Williams, 1979). Shaper's work on the Samburu (Shaper, 1962; Shaper *et al.,* 1969), however, showed *lower* blood cholesterol and phospholipid levels in soldiers in whom blood pressure was higher than in native warriors who consume between 2 and 15 pints of milk per person per day. Data from Indian railway workers (Malhotra, 1970) is also contradictory.

Protein

Hypotension is a characteristic clinical sign of protein-energy malnutrition and a reduction of blood pressure is an early event when primates are fed a low protein diet (Fiorotto, 1980). The mechanism responsible for this effect is unknown, although marked alterations in renal blood flow are an early feature of the response to a low protein.

In unacculturated peoples protein intakes (which are generally poorly documented) may well be below the FAO/WHO recommended intakes, but above the levels which lead to clinically apparent malnutrition. A role for increased protein intake in inducing the rise in blood pressure following acculturation cannot therefore be ruled out.

Stress

The idea that the stresses and strains of the western way of life cause hypertension has been put forward several times (Foster, 1927; Tung, 1927; Donnison, 1929; Saunders, 1932; Nye, 1937; Kaminer and Lutz, 1960). Pickering (Couvee, 1962) considers that Bushmen are not subjected to the stress of making decisions because "so much is laid down by ritual and taboo" and that this is a more plausible reason for their lack of hypertension than the absence of salt in their diet. The objective measurement of stress across linguistic and cultural barriers is difficult and has not been undertaken in conjunction with studies of blood pressure. It has been claimed (Truswell, 1977) that, since the prevalence of hypertension in negroes in the USA is higher in rural than urban areas, then the stresses of urban life are not a factor in the development of the disease. This is also true of Japan (Schroeder, 1958), but mortality data from England and Wales show the opposite trend with standardized mortality ratios for hypersensitive diseases in both men and women consistently higher in conurbations than in rural areas (Offices of Population Censuses and Surveys, 1969–73). There are some indications that noise, particularly from low flying aircraft, is hypertensinogenic in man (Ettema and Zielhuis, 1977). When exposed experimentally to noise adults show a rise in blood pressure; hypertension is more frequently encountered in groups subjected chronically to the noise of low flying aircraft.

In animals, elevated blood pressure has been produced by stressful situations such as food–shock conflict (Friedman and Iwai, 1977). Strains of rats sensitive to the development of hypertension on a high salt diet (Dahl, 1972) are rendered moderately hypersensitive by exposure to a food–shock conflict even in the absence of a high salt diet. The resistant rats show no rise in blood pressure in this situation. When sensitive strains of rats are simultaneously exposed to a moderately high salt diet (2% NaCl) and a stressful situation, the level of hypertension is greater than that seen with stress and a low salt intake, and very much greater than that seen with a 2% NaCl diet in the absence of stress (Friedman and Iwai, 1977).

The conclusion from animal experiments such as these is that stress can act synergistically with sodium in the production of hypertension but that, in the absence of sodium sensitivity, its effect is slight.

Potassium

A protective role for potassium has been argued strongly by Meneeley and Batterbee (1976). Certainly unprocessed vegetable diets low in sodium are also high in potassium and the processing and cooking of these foods decreases the potassium content and increases that of sodium (Meneeley and Batterbee, 1976). The Yanomamo, who show no rise in blood pressure with age and have no hypertension, excrete large quantities of potassium (200 mEq/24 h) with a small sodium output (1 mEq/24 h) (Sasaki et al., 1959). The presence of lower blood pressures and lower stroke mortality, despite high salt consumption, in Japanese from the Aomori prefecture, has been attributed to the simultaneous ingestion of large amounts of potassium in the form of apples (Sasaki, 1962).

Animal experiments have been cited which support a protective effect of potassium in the face of a high sodium intake. Meneeley et al. (1957) have ameliorated the hypertensive effect of salt in rats by feeding large quantities of potassium. The possibility that a high potassium intake may counteract any hypertensive effect of a high sodium intake could be of considerable pulic health importance.

Chronic infection

The possibility that chronic infection in unacculturated groups is instrumental in keeping blood pressures low has been mentioned by several early authors and discussed by Fries (1976). Maddocks (1967), in his study of five Melanesian populations, states that his "findings are at least consistent with the hypothesis that chronic infection tends to keep blood pressures low". Malaria and chronic infestations are prevalent in other groups without hypertension (Burns-Cox and Maclean, 1970) but this is not true of all (Page *et al.,* 1974; Srinivasan *et al.,* 1980; Donnison, 1929). It is curious that in taking values of blood pressure found in their own cultures as norms, investigators have felt compelled to attribute the absence of hypertension to the presence of disease.

Sucrose

Little attention has been give to dietary sucrose as a possible agent promoting hypertension. However, recent studies in spider monkeys suggest that when 38% of the dietary energy was consumed as dietary sucrose rather than complex carbohydrate, then the salt-induced increase in blood pressure was enhanced (Table X). These results conform with earlier results in rodents, but the mechanisms underlying the interaction are obscure: they may involve alterations in sodium handling by the kidney or more complex interactions on the sympathomimetic system, since Young and Landsberg (1978) have found a decrease in catecholamine turnover on starvation, with a restitution to normal with sucrose feeding alone. Data in humans are less clear. Jung *et al.* (1979) found that a reduction in carbohydrate intake (including sucrose) in normotensive obese women led to a prompt fall in blood pressure independently of any change in sodium intake; the fall in blood pressure was associated with a fall in hydroxy-methoxymandelic acid excretion, the main excretory product of catecholamine metabolisms. Thus

Table X

Blood pressure and diet (Srinivasan *et al.,* 1980).

Dietary group	Increase (mmHg)[a]			
	Systolic		Diastolic	
Control	8·9	2·4	5·6	1·9
3% NaCl	19·4	2·5	6·7	2·1
3% NaCl + 38% energy as sucrose	24·0	2·9	10·4	1·4

[a]Expressed as differences from basal periods of observation with 16 triplicate readings on six spider monkeys fed each type of diet. The increase in systolic and diastolic blood pressure compared with the control dietary values was at least $p < 0.01$.

there is evidence that carbohydrate intake may affect blood pressure in man and the exacerbation by sucrose of the hypertensive response to salt in monkeys suggests the possibility of a specific effect of sucrose.

The concept of excess energy intake leading to enhanced activity of the sympathomimetic system is an important one which may, in part, explain the association between obesity and hypertension and the beneficial effects on blood pressure of weight reduction.

Calcium

There have been many studies which have looked at the relationship between sudden death from cardiovascular disease and the "hardness" of the drinking water. Most investigators find that the "harder" the water, the lower the death rate from cardiovascular disease, including hypertension (Sharrett and Feinlab, 1975), yet no pathophysiological link has been proposed between calcium intake and cardiovascular disease.

Recent studies by Ayachi (1979) show that doubling the dietary calcium of spontaneously hypertensive rats to $2 \cdot 5\%$ of the diet reduces their blood pressure and leads to a greater urinary output of calcium, potassium and sodium. Food intakes were not recorded but the body weights of the animals were similar so that the suppression of blood pressure by dietary calcium was apparently not via an effect on food intake. Since the 24-hour potassium (K^+) and sodium (Na^+) output was unusually increased on the high calcium diet, the absorption and faecal excretion of sodium and potassium must have been different if food intakes were the same and the animals in a steady state. A state of functional hypoparathyroidism may also have contributed to the lower blood pressure. These animal experiments show the need for caution before dietary factors unconnected with the usual hypotheses linking diet and hypertension are dismissed as of little likely significance.

The impact of hypertension on health

This has already been discussed in detail in relation to the development in ischaemic heart disease and the relation of hypertension to the incidence of stroke is well established. It should, however, be noted that in the UK we know little about the prevalence rates of hypertension in different parts of Britain. Some indication that these may differ is suggested by the marked variation in the minority rates for men and women dying of cerebrovascular disease in this country (Table XI). Whether these differences relate to variable rates of hypertension or other factors, e.g. vitamin C intakes (see Fig. 7) is unknown, but certainly warrants further investigation.

Table XI

Mortality from cerebrovascular disease at ages 15−64 by sex
and regional hospital board in England and Wales, 1970−2.
(From Occupational Mortality Tables by area.)

		Standardized mortality rates	
		Men	Women
1.	Newcastle	127	119
2.	Leeds	106	103
3.	Sheffield	102	99
4.	East Anglia	82	96
5.	N.W. Metropolitan (London)	76	81
6.	N.E. Metropolitan (London)	78	80
7.	S.E. Metropolitan (London)	84	94
8.	S.W. Metropolitan (London)	84	82
9.	Wessex	86	86
10.	Oxford	87	84
11.	South Western	96	96
12.	Birmingham	128	118
13.	Liverpool	110	108
14.	Manchester	128	125
15.	Wales	110	118

Obesity

Unlike the problems of ischaemic heart disease and hypertension, the idea
that obesity is a diet-related condition is much easier to accept. Yet an
examination of the dietary data relating to obesity could be considered more
confusing than the information linking diets to the development of
atherosclerosis or high blood pressure.

Obesity affects 15−25% of the middle-aged and elderly populations of
the UK (see Table XII). An even larger proportion of adults is overweight,
with 55−65% of the population with weights in excess of that considered
optimal in terms of life expectancy as deduced from the data collected by
the Metropolitan Life Insurance Company of New York (James, 1976).
Obesity leads to a marked increase in mortality and morbidity and the risk
of developing complications of obesity, e.g. diabetes mellitus, gallstone
disease and osteoarthritis, increases progressively with increasing degrees of
overweight. If obese individuals return to a normal weight and are able to
maintain this weight then their life expectancy also returns to normal
(Dublin, 1953). The problem of obesity therefore constitutes a major public
health problem in this country.

Table XII

Prevalence of overweight and obesity (%) in randomly sampled
populations in the UK

	Below desirable range	Within desirable range	Borderline	Overweight	Obesity
Based on medium frame size[a]					
Women	16·2	24·2	22·2	14·4	22·4
Men	14·7	19·9	27·1	21·2	17·1
Based on all three frame sizes[a]					
Women	10·3	50·9	17·2	9·6	12·0
Men	8·2	50·0	24·1	11·5	6·2
Total numbers of subjects: 2343 women, 2057 men					

[a]Upper limit of desirable weight taken for calculating cut-off points for
overweight and obesity and lower limits for calculating underweights.

Data on the prevalence of obesity in children in affluent societies suggests
that it is an increasing problem, although the criteria used to define obesity
are not readily standardized (Forbes, 1973; James, 1976). In the USA the
Ten-State Nutrition Survey (1968–70) showed that as many as 24% of 16-to
17-year-old white boys could be classified as obese on the basis of a high
triceps skinfold thickness. Black boys of equivalent age have a lower
prevalence by the same criteria, although it is often overlooked that the
triceps skinfold thickness may be much smaller in negro children of
equivalent weight for height than white children; sub-scapular skinfold
measurements are a better index of body fat (Robson *et al.,* 1971).

The prevalence of obesity varies considerably from country to country
but where sequential studies have been undertaken in a specific area, e.g.
Czechoslovakia (Hejda, 1978) then over a 15-year period the prevalence of
obesity in 20-year-old boys appears to have more than doubled, the secular
change being much less obvious in young women. The differences between
the prevalence of obesity in boys and girls and between men and women,
and the differences in prevalence among the social classes have been
emphasized by Garn and his co-workers in their analysis of the relative
importance of heredity and environment in determining the onset of obesity
(Garn and Clark, 1976; Garn *et al.,* 1976). A collection of data from a
number of studies in the UK (James, 1976) shows that the prevalence falls
steadily from a rate of about 35% at the age of about 1 year to 7% at the
age of 6–11 years, after which time there is a further increase at a time when
preferential fat deposition is well recognized (Dugdale and Payne, 1975;
Garn and Clark, 1976).

Over the last 40 years the average body fat content of the adult population in the UK has increased by about 10% and it is therefore likely that the prevalence of obesity in adults has also increased. This change probably relates to a number of environmental factors: to changes in the economic and social environment and to a reduction in the amount of physical activity undertaken by adults. Physical exertion at work has been reduced with the mechanization of industrial processes, housework is less time-consuming and less physically demanding and the increased use of the private motor car by a larger proportion of the population has also contributed to a fall in the amount of exercise taken by adults. However, apart from the period of food rationing during and after the Second World War, there has been no reduction in the calculated average intake of food energy until a decline began in the early 1970s (National Food Survey Committee). Given the fall in energy expenditure, it would not be surprising if the average weight of the population had increased as subjects adapt to the relative excess of food intake.

Although there has been little change in the total amount of energy consumed per head from 1930 to 1970, there have been substantial changes in the source of the food energy. Sugar consumption (Davidson *et al.,* 1975) and alcohol intake have increased and the total fat intake may also have risen, although the basis for these calculations is now disputed (Trenchard, 1977). The fractions of energy derived from fat has increased substantially. There has also been a gradual decline in the intake of total dietary fibre (Southgate *et al.,* 1978) and a change in the proportions coming from different sources; there has been a small increase in vegetable fibre intake and a slow fall in cereal fibre consumption. Statistics on the body weight of adults in Britain are not available to allow an analysis of the relationships between changes in the pattern of food consumed and changes in body weight – analyses conducted on data collected immediately after the Second World War related to the relationship of weight to total energy intake only (Harries and Hollingworth, 1953).

There has been a change in the pattern of eating with a fall in the number of people eating breakfast and an increased emphasis on the evening meal (National Food Survey Committee, Annual Report, 1977). A reduction in the number of meals consumed each day has been linked with an increased likelihood of gaining weight (Fabry, 1973), but this is not backed up by careful studies with whole-body calorimetry on young men receiving their food energy in either two or six meals per day. They had an equivalent energy output in the calorimeter on both regimes (Dallosso and James, 1981).

Evidence will be presented below to show that the source of the dietary energy does affect energy utilization and energy expenditure.

Energy balance and obesity

If food energy is ingested and absorbed in amounts which exceed the energy used by the body, then the excess energy is retained mainly as fat. The amount of energy needed by the body varies considerably from person to person so that some children or adults may normally use twice the amount of energy ingested by other individuals of equivalent size (Widdowson, 1962; Rose and Williams, 1961). These differences in energy requirement do not relate simply to differences in physical activity because there are also substantial differences in the basal energy requirement for maintaining normal processes and in the individual responses to food. If an individual consumes more energy than he needs then the body adapts to compensate for the energy imbalance. The ability to compensate varies markedly: some adults who normally need 12·5 MJ (3000 kcals) can be overfed until after several weeks they attain a new state of energy balance on an intake of 20·9 MJ (5000 kcals), this adaptation being accompanied by an increase in body weight of only 10% (Sims *et al.,* 1973). Other less fortunate subjects cannot compensate so well and readily gain weight.

Given this ability of the body to buffer changes in energy intake, it is perhaps not surprising that despite the reduced activity of the population there have been only small secular changes in the average body fat of individuals. During an adult's lifetime a 500 kJ (120 kcal) difference between energy input and output would, on a cumulative basis, lead to marked changes in body weight; these changes are relatively slow and represent discrepancies of only 2% of the total energy turnover per day.

Energy intake in obesity

Investigations on the food intake of obese individuals do not show that they eat more than their slim counterparts. These findings have been obtained in overweight babies, obese adolescents and obese adults. Sixty-three obese women were studied by McCarthy (1966), with a seven-day food diary; the obese ingested (mean ± SD) 7·85 ± 2·23 MJ/day (1884 ± 534 kcal/day), whereas the intake of 26 normal weight controls was 8·24 ± 2·0 MJ/day (1978 ± 479 kcal/day). Maxfield and Konishi (1966) investigated 25 obese women, paired by age with non-obese women, and again found similar intakes in the two groups: 7·8 ± 3·64 MJ/day (1871 ± 873 kcal/day) in the obese, and 8·28 ± 2·93 MJ/day (1986 ± 704 kcal/day) in the lean. Social class does not affect this comparison since Durnin *et al.* (1974) found a consistently lower energy intake in the fattest adolescent girls of all social groups compared with similar aged non-obese girls from the same background. Even studies on obese and non-obese infants show similar energy intakes (Sveger *et al.*, 1975).

Physical activity in obesity

In most individuals in Britain and in many children, physical activity accounts for about 20% of the daily energy expenditure. The energy cost of daily activity is difficult to assess because it is very variable both between individuals and in the same individual from time to time. Using cinematography, Bullen *et al.* (1964) reported that although obese adolescent girls spend a similar amount of time at physical activity as lean girls, the degree of movement was less in the obese. Nevertheless, the additional energy cost of moving in the obese girls was not assessed so that it is likely that the total work output was at least the same if not more than that in the slim girls since the energy cost of physical activity shows an increase in a linear fashion with the subject's weight (Miller and Parsonage, 1975). As yet there is little evidence to suggest that some feature of physical activity is the key to the development and maintenance of the obese state.

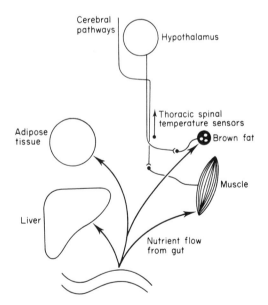

Figure 11 Dietary intake and thermogenesis. Nutrients from the diet are distributed to all tissues of the body, but dietary fat can be used as a fuel for brown adipose tissue (brown fat) which is considered to be less active in familial obesity and therefore less able to dissipate energy as heat from dietary fat.

In searching for any dietary factors which may relate to obesity, it is now becoming clear that the thermogenic response to mixed meals is different in slim and obese individuals (Shetty *et al.,* 1981). Responses to starch and protein seem to be similar, however, and the principal difference appears to be in the response to dietary fat.

Figure 11 summarizes our current view of the mechanism whereby dietary fat leads to less heat production in obese people than thin individuals. The concept that brown adipose tissue may be the key to the difference between lean and obese individuals depends on two pieces of evidence. First is the demonstration that the responsiveness of this tissue is the key to the metabolic basis of obesity in one strain of genetically obese animals, the ob/ob mouse (Thurlby and Trayhurn, 1980). Secondly, obese adults from fat families display similar responses to the hormone noradrenaline (which mediates the non-shivering thermogenic response in the body) to those seen in the ob/ob mouse. Brown adipose tissue depends for its fuel on the provision of external sources of fatty acid, or, in their absence, on a high synthetic rate of fatty acids from glucose. The newborn animal has brown adipose tissue distributed widely in the body and there are high activities of the enzyme lipoprotein lipase in the brown adipose tissue to channel fuel into an organ which is crucial to survival in the early period of life. It would not be surprising, therefore, to find in adults that the inflow of dietary fat would lead to differential heating effects depending on the degree to which the brown adipose tissue remains in a preserved and responsive state in adult life.

Since obesity is recognized to be a familial condition, we need to recogize that these families may be displaying obesity selectively as a response to an environment in which there is a relative excess of food with a high fat content. Children of obese parents, before they become fat, have a lower food intake than normal and their total energy output is also 20% below that of similar weight children from thin families (Griffiths and Payne, 1976). These children have a reduced need for energy to maintain their body weight and the normal intake observed in so many obese adults therefore reflects an excess intake for their individual needs.

Here, then, in obesity we find the same problem of an interaction between environmental and genetic susceptibility. Figure 12 displays this interaction by showing how the prevalence of obesity in a community will depend on the provision of an abundant, varied and palatable high-fat diet. In this environment there will also be an increase in the prevalence of obesity with age either because of the progressive decline in physical activity or because of a more fundamental metabolic reason. Within a single society, however, the individuals affected by the environmental conditions will be those most genetically susceptible and with a lower metabolic response to fatty foods, i.e. reduced postprandial thermogenesis.

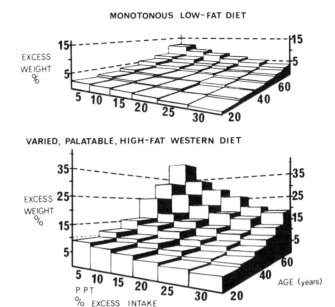

Figure 12 Social and constitutional interactions in determining obesity. PPT: postprandial thermogenesis. This is a hypothetical scheme based on Borhani (1977).

The emphasis in this section has been on the importance of the individual's susceptibility to obesity because the usual response to the problem of obesity is to assume the overwhelming importance of social and psychological factors in its determination. In the other conditions discussed —ischaemic heart disease and hypertension—physicians have readily accepted the genetic evidence but sought to reject the environmental contribution. ALL THREE DISEASES CAN, HOWEVER, BE CONSIDERED AS THE OUTCOME OF DIFFERING DEGREES OF ENVIRONMENTAL INFLUENCES ON AN INDIVIDUAL'S GENETICALLY DETERMINED METABOLIC RESPONSE TO DIET.

Colon cancer

Cancer of the colon will be considered as one example of a more difficult problem in the analysis of dietary patterns and disease states. In this condition we are having to deal with a much less common disease than the three others considered so far and one where there is no familial aggregation of cases except in the specific condition of polyposis coli. Nevertheless, we need to recognize the increasing evidence that environmental factors and probably diet do contribute, even though we are far less clear about the mechanisms involved.

Large bowel cancer is the second most common cancer leading to death in England and Wales (Table XIII) and there is evidence that it is becoming

Table XIII

Cancer incidence in the Birmingham region
1968−72.

| | % Total cancers | |
	Males	Females
Bronchus and trachea	32	6
Gut		
stomach	8	3
colon	5	6
rectum	5	3
Hormone-dependent		
prostate	3	
testis	1	
breast		30
uterus		5
Cervix		8
Bladder	6	2
Non-melanotic skin	12	8
Other	26	22

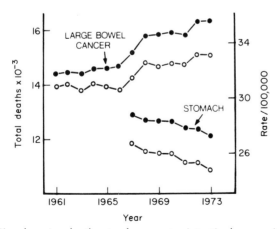

Figure 13   The changing death rates from gastro-intestinal cancer in England and Wales. Total deaths per annum ●-● ; Death rate per 100,000 of the population o-o. Calculations are based on the Registrar General's Annual Reviews (Cummings, 1976).

increasingly common (Fig. 13). Armstrong and Doll (1975) related the mortality rate of colon cancer to the estimated food consumption per capita in different countries. The dietary data are a poor basis for comparison but nevertheless it is apparent that there are marked variations in the cancer rate around the world. Armstrong and Doll found a high correlation between the consumption of animal protein and fats and the mortality from colon cancer; there was a negative correlation with cereal consumption. First-order partial correlation coefficients were calculated for the various food groups and it became clear that the best correlation was found for animal protein, the negative association with cereal consumption no longer proving statistically significant.

Migrants tend, on moving to their new country, to take on the cancer pattern of their host country. This is shown, for example, in Japanese migrants who, in the USA have higher cancer rates which match those of American whites more closely than those of Japanese living in Japan (Haenszel and Kurihara, 1968).

Hill and his colleagues proposed that dietary fat might be the key to colon carcinogenesis by promoting an increase in the concentration of colonic bile acids which might then serve as carcinogens or co-carcinogens (Aries *et al.*, 1969). Hill then went on to show that groups in Africa, Asia, Europe and North America had increasing concentrations of dihydroxycholanic acid in the faeces and a high anaerobe to aerobe ratio in proportion to the increase in the cancer rates of those countries (Hill *et al.*, 1971). More detailed studies in Hong Kong also showed differences in faecal steroid concentrations which corresponded to the differing cancer rates in low, middle and high income groups (Crowther *et al.*, 1976).

Recently we have also undertaken a more detailed study of dietary patterns and colon cancer in Scandinavia as part of a collaborative exercise co-ordinated by the International Agency for Research on Cancer (I.A.R.C., 1977). In Copenhagen there is a higher rate of colon cancer than in rural Finland, yet the Finns consume more fat and animal protein. On this occasion, however, the faecal steroid concentrations were not different in the two countries. More recent unpublished studies are in keeping with the Hill hypothesis, provided it is modified to include an important role for dietary fibre which appears to exert a dominating effect on colonic microbial metabolism.

On this basis Cummings has proposed a scheme to explain the interactions of diet on colon carcinogenesis as illustrated in Fig. 14. To substantiate those observations will require a great deal more work with a combination of metabolic–epidemiological and physiological studies. These approaches signify a new way of looking at the diseases of affluence which is very different from the traditional one. Without a clear mechanism

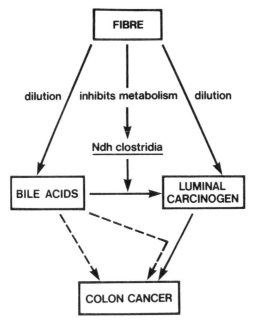

Figure 14   Potential protective mechanisms of dietary fibre in the development of colon cancer (Cummings, 1976).

to explain a disease process, scientists tend to neglect general epidemiological associations. However, by detailed studies with sequential efforts to test hypotheses relating diet to colonic metabolism, we should come closer to understanding the key environmental factors responsible for cancer of the colon.

Conclusions

No attempt has been made to give a comprehensive account of the many prevalent diseases in which dietary factors are now being implicated nor has there been an exhaustive analysis of the evidence for the nutritional basis of a single disease. Instead the emphasis has been on displaying how one can piece together the evidence from many different types of study to show how in western societies one needs to recognize the important interaction between environmental factors and genetic susceptibility in determining which members of a community succumb to different diseases. The evidence that diet affects a number of important metabolic processes of relevance to disease states is overwhelming and this must be recognized even when we are uncertain of the precise mechanism responsible for obesity, ischaemic heart disease or many other conditions.

The present article is not an attempt to make a case for intervening on a population basis to alter the dietary pattern of the community. A decision that such action is necessary is a separate issue from the scientific case for the role of diet in the aetiology of disease. Scientists well versed in the critical appraisal of experimental data will require "proof" of connections between diet and disease before they feel comfortable in recommending any changes. Those involved in public policy-making, however, have to act on the basis of incomplete evidence and their appreciation of the quality of evidence may be very different. The present chapter attempts to highlight the rapidly accumulating evidence which shows that nutritional disease should no longer be considered simply in terms of protein, vitamin or mineral deficiencies. Nutritional research must now call on many different disciplines if the role of nutritional factors in the prevalence of disease is to be assessed adequately, but current evidence already suggests that nutritional research should be at the forefront of attempts to explain many of the prevalent diseases which are at present a major economic burden on the community.

Acknowledgement

We would like to thank Mrs Miriam Rundle for her painstaking help with the preparation and typing of the manuscript.

References

Acheson, R. M. and Williams, D. R. R. (1979) "Epidemiology of Strokes: Some Unanswered Questions". Proceedings of Symposium on Neuro-Epidemiology at the Medical Society of London. Pitmans, London.

Alexander, J. K. (1975) Interactions of hyperlipidaemia, hypertension and obesity as coronary risk factors. *Triangle,* **14,** 1.

Anderson, G. F., Lifschutz, C. and Friis-Lasen, B. (1979) Dietary habits and serum lipids during first 4 years of life. *Acta Paediatrica Scandinavica,* **68,** 165.

Aries, V. C., Crowther, J. S., Draser, B. S., Hill, M. J. and Williams, R. E. O. (1969) Bacteria and the aetiology of cancer of the large bowel. *Gut,* **10,** 334.

Armstrong, B. and Doll, R. (1975) Environmental factors and cancer incidence and mortality in different countries, with special reference to dietary practices. *International Journal of Cancer,* **15,** 617.

Ayachi, S. (1979) Increased dietary calcium lowers blood pressure in the spontaneously hypertensive rat. *Metabolism,* **28,** 1234.

Berglund, E. and Wilhelmsen, L. (1975) Factors related to blood pressure in a general population sample of Swedish men. *Acta Medica Scandinavica,* **198,** 291.

Bianchi, G., Fox, V., Di Francesco, Giovannetti, A. M. and Pagetti, D. (1974). Blood pressure changes produced by kidney cross transplantation between spontaneously hypertensive rats (SHR) and normotensive rats (NR). *Clinical Science and Molecular Medicine,* **47,** 435.

Borhani, N. O. (1977) Primary prevention of coronary heart disease: a critique. *American Journal of Cardiology,* **40,** 251.

Brown, J., Bourke, G. J., Gearty, G. F., Finnegan, A., Hill, M., Heffernan-Fox, F. C., Fitzgerald, D. E., Kennedy, J., Childers, R. W., Jessop, W. T. E., Toulson, M. F., Latham, M. C., Cronin, S., McCann, M. B., Clancy, R. E., Gore, I., Stoudt, H. W., Hegsted, D. M. and Stone, F. J. (1970) Nutritional and epidemiological factors related to heart disease. *World Review of Nutrition and Dietetics,* **12,**1.

Bullen, B. A., Reed, R. B. and Mayer, J. (1964) Physical activity of obese and non-obese adolescent girls appraised by motion picture sampling. *American Journal of Clinical Nutrition* **14,** 211.

Burns-Cox, C. J. and Maclean, J. D. (1970) Splenomegaly and blood pressure in an Orang Asli community in West Malaysia. *American Heart Journal,* **80,** 718.

Burstyn, P. G. and Firth, W. R. (1975) Effects of three fat-enriched diets on the arterial pressure of rabbits. *Cardiovascular Research,* **9,** 807.

Byington, R., Dyer, A. R., Garside, D., Liu, K., Moss, D., Stamler, J. and Tsong, Y. (1979) Recent trends of major coronary risk factors and C.H.D. mortality in the United States and other industrialized countries. *In* "Proceedings of Conference on the decline in coronary heart disease mortality", R. J. Havlik and M. Feinlab (eds). U.S.D. H.E.W. N.I.H. Publication 79, p.340.

Clarke, W. R., Woolson, R., Schrott, H., Wiebe, D. and Lauer, R. M. (1976) Tracking of blood pressure serum lipids and obesity in children: the Muscatine Study. *Circulation,* **54** (Suppl. II), 23.

Committee of Principal Investigators (1978) A cooperative trial in the prevention of ischaemic heart disease using clofibrate. *British Heart Journal,* **40,** 1069.

Committee of Principal Investigators (1980) WHO cooperative trial on primary prevention of ischaemic heart disease using clofibrate to lower serum cholesterol: mortality follow-up. *Lancet,* **ii,** 379.

Couvee, L. M. J. (1962) The nutritional condition of the Kapauku in the central highlands of W. New Guinea. Discussion by G. Pickering. *Tropical and Geographical Medicine,* **14**

Crowther, J. S., Draser, B. S., Hill, M. J., MacLennan, R., Magnin, D., Peach, S. and Teoh-Chan, C. H. (1976) Faecal steroids and bacteria and large bowel cancer in Hong Kong by socio-economic groups. *British Journal of Cancer,* **34,** 191.

Cummings, J. H. (1976) Dietary fibre and large bowel cancer. *In* "A Symposium on Dietary Fibre", p.40. Reckitt and Colman, London.

Dahl, L. K. (1961) Possible role of chronic excess salt consumption in the pathogenesis of essential hypertension. *American Journal of Cardiology,* **8,**571.

Dahl, L. K. (1972) Salt and hypertension. *American Journal of Clinical Nutrition,* **25,** 231.

Dahl, L. K., Heine, M. and Thompson, K. (1974) Genetic influences of the kidney on blood pressure. Evidence from chronic renal homografts in rats with opposite predispositions to hypotension. *Circulation Research,* **40,** 94.

Dallosso, H. and James, W. P. T. (1981) Feeding frequency and human energy expenditure levels measured continuously for 24 hrs. *In* "Recent Advances in Obesity Research", A. N. Howard (ed.) (in press).

Davidson, S., Passmore, R., Brock, J. F. and Truswell, A. S. (1975) "Human Nutrition and Dietetics", p. 216. Churchill Livingstone, Edinburgh.

DHSS (1974) Report of the Advisory Panel of the Committee on Medical Aspects of Food Policy (Nutrition) on Diet in relation to Cardiovascular and Cerebrovascular Disease, No. 7. HMSO, London.

Donnison, C. P. (1929) Blood pressure in the African native. *Lancet,* i, 6.

Dublin, L. I. (1953) Relation of obesity to longevity. *New England Journal of Medicine,* **248,** 971.

Dugdale, A. E. and Payne, P. R. (1975) Pattern of fat and lean tissue deposition in children. *Nature,* **256,** 725.

Durnin, J. V. G. A., Lonergan, M. E., Good, J. and Ewan, A. (1974) A cross-sectional nutritional and anthropometric study, with an interval of 7 years, on 611 young adolescent schoolchildren. *British Journal of Nutrition,* **32,** 169.

Dyerberg, J., Bang, H. O., Stofferson, E., Moncada, S. and Vane, J. R. (1978) Eicosapentaenoic acid and prevention of thrombosis and atherosclerosis. *Lancet,* **ii,** 117.

Eating and Drinking Habits. Report on a Food Survey 1977. Heublein International Management Corporation.

Ettema, J. H. and Zielhuis, R. L. (1977) Health effects of exposure to noise, particularly aircraft noise. *International Archives of Occupational and Environmental Health,* **40,** 163.

Fabry, P. (1973) Food intake pattern and energy balance. *In* "Energy Balance in Man", M. Apfelbaum (ed.), p. 297. Masson, Paris.

Fiorotto, M. (1980) Studies on oedema formation in experimental protein-energy malnutrition. Ph.D. Thesis, Cambridge University.

Forbes, G. B. (1973) Prevalence of obesity in childhood. *In* "Obesity in Perspective", G. A. Bray (ed.). DHEW Publ. No. NIH 75−708 p. 205.

Foster, J. H. (1927) Blood pressure of foreigners in China. *Archives of Internal Medicine,* **40,** 38.

Foster, J. H. (1930) Practice of medicine in China and New England with observations on hypertension. *New England Journal of Medicine,* **203,** 1073.

Friedman, R. and Iwai, J. (1977) Dietary sodium, psychic stress and genetic predisposition to experimental hypertension. *Proceedings of the Society for Experimental Biology and Medicine,* **155,** 449.

Fries, E. D. (1976) Salt, volume and the prevention of hypertension. *Circulation,* **53,** 589.

Fuster, V., Bowie, E. J. W., Lewis, J. C., Fass, D. N., Owen, C. A. Jr and Brown, A. L. (1978) Resistance to arteriosclerosis in pigs with von Willebrand's disease. Spontaneous and high cholesterol diet-induced arteriosclerosis. *Journal of Clinical Investigation,* **61,** 722.

Garay, R. P. and Meyer, P. (1979) A new test showing abnormal net Na^+ and K^+ fluxes in erythrocytes of essential hypertensive patients. *Lancet,* i, 349.

Garn, S. M. and Clark, D. C. (1976) Trends in fatness and the origins of obesity. *Paediatrics,* **57,** 443.

Garn, S. M., Bailey, S. M., Cole, P. E. and Higgins, I. T. T. (1977) Level of education, level of income and level of fatness in adults. *American Journal of Clinical Nutrition,* **30,** 721.

Gleibermann, L. (1973) Blood pressure and dietary salt in human populations. *Ecology of Food and Nutrition,* **2,** 143.

Glueck, C. J., Gartside, P., Fallat, R. W., Sielski, J. and Steiner, P.M. (1976) Longevity syndromes. Familial hypobeta and familial hyperalpha lipoproteinaemia. *Journal of Laboratory and Clinical Medicine,* **88,** 941.

Glueck, C. J., Gartside, P. S., Steiner, P. M., Miller, M., Todhunter, T., Haaf, J., Pucke, M., Terrana, M., Fallat, R. W. and Kashyap, M. L. (1977) Hyperalpha- and hypobeta-lipoproteinemia in octogenarian kindreds. *Atherosclerosis,* **27,** 387.

Griffiths, M. and Payne, P. R. (1976) Energy expenditure in small children of obese and non-obese parents. *Nature,* **260,** 698.

Haenszel, W. and Kurihara, M. (1968) Studies of Japanese migrants. I. Mortality from cancer and other diseases among Japanese in the United States. *Journal of the National Cancer Institute,* **49,** 43.

Harker, L. A., Ross, R., Slichter, S. J. and Scott, C. R. (1976) Homocystine-induced arteriosclerosis. The role of endothelial cell injury and platelet response in its genesis. *Journal of Clinical Investigation,* **58,** 731.

Harries, J. M. and Hollingsworth, D. F. (1953) Food supply, body weight and activity in Great Britain 1943–9. *British Medical Journal,* **1,** 75.

Havlik, R. J. and Feinlab, M. (eds.) (1979) "Proceedings of the Conference on the decline in coronary heart disease mortality", U.S.D. H.E.W. N.I.H. Publication 79, p. 1610.

Heart Detection and Follow-up Program (1979) Five-year findings of the hypertension detection and follow-up program. I. Reduction in mortality of persons with high blood pressure, including mild hypertension; II. Mortality by Race, Sex and Age. *Journal of the American Medical Association,* **242,** 2562, 2572.

Hedja, S. (1978) Problems of obesity in Czechoslovakia and comparable countries. *In* Marabou Symposium "Why Obesity?", H. Mogren (ed.). Suppl.Nr 15 til Naringsforskning, argang 22, p. 46.

Hegsted, D. M., McGandy, R. B., Myers, M. L. and Stare, F. J. (1965) Quantitative effects of dietary fat on serum cholesterol in man. *American Journal of Clinical Nutrition,* **17,** 281.

Hill, M. J., Drasar, B. S., Aries, V. C., Crowther, J. S., Hawksworth, G. M. and Williams, R. E. O. (1971) Bacteria and aetiology of cancer of large bowel. *Lancet,* **i,** 95.

Hipsley, E. H. and Clements, F. W. (1947) "Report of the New Guineas Nutrition Survey Expedition". Department of External Territories, Canberra.

Iacono, J. M., Marshall, M. W., Dougherty, R. M., Wheeler, M. A., Mackin, J. F. and Canary, J. J. (1975) Reduction in blood pressure associated with high polyunsaturated fat diets that reduce blood cholesterol in man. *Preventive Medicine,* **4,** 426.

International Agency of Research on Cancer Microecology Group (1977) Dietary fibre, transit time, faecal bacteria, steroids and colon cancer in two Scandinavian populations. *Lancet,* **ii,** 207.

James, W. P. T. (1976) "Research on Obesity". A Report of the DHSS/MRC Group. London, HMSO.

Joossens, J. V. (1973) Salt and hypertension, water hardness and cardiovascular death rates. *Triangle,* 12, 9.

Joossens, J. V. (1980) Trends in cardiovascular mortality. *Acta Cardiologica,* (in press).

Joosens, J. V., Willems, J., Claessens, J., Claes, J. and Lissens, W. (1970) Sodium and hypertension. *In* "Nutrition and Cardiovascular Diseases". Proceedings of the 7th International Meeting of the Centro Studi Lipidi Alimentari-Biologia and Clinica Della Nutrizione—Fondazione Sasso Rimini, Sept. 25/26.

Kaminer, B. and Lutz, W. P. (1960) Blood pressure in Bushmen of the Kalahari Desert. *Circulation,* 22, 289.

Kato, H., Tillotson, J., Nichaman, M., Rhoads, G. G. and Hamilton, H. B. (1973) Epidemiologic studies of coronary heart disease and stroke in Japanese men living in Japan, Hawaii and California: serum lipids and diet. *American Journal of Epidemiology,* 97, 372.

Keys, A. (1980) "Seven Countries: A Multivariate Analysis of Death and Coronary Heart Disease". Harvard University Press, Cambridge, Mass. and London.

Keys, A. and Kimura, N. (1970) Diets of middle-aged farmers in Japan. *American Journal of Clinical Nutrition,* 23, 2, 212.

Keys, A., Anderson, J. T. and Grande, F. (1959) Serum cholesterol in man: diet fat and intrinsic responsiveness. *Circulation,* 19, 201.

Kwiterovich, P. D., Levy, R. I. and Frederickson, D. S. (1973) Neonatal diagnosis of familial type II hyperlipoproteinaemia. *Lancet,* i, 118.

Johnson, B. C., Epstein, F. H. and Kjelsberg, M. O. (1965) Distributions and familial studies of blood pressure and serum cholesterol levels in a total community—Tecumseh, Michigan. *Journal of Chronic Diseases,* 18, 147.

Jung, R. T., Shetty, P. S., Barrand, M., Callingham, B. A. and James, W. P. T. (1979) Role of catecholamines in hypotensive response to dieting. *British Medical Journal,* 1, 12.

Lauer, R. M., Clarke, W., Reiter, M. A. and Schrott, H. (1977) Coronary risk factors in children: the Muscatine Study. *In* "Proceedings of the Workshop on Atherosclerosis and the Child", p.14. Department of Human Nutrition, Agricultural University, Wageningen, Netherlands.

Liu, K., Cooper, R., McKeever, J., McKeever, P., Byington, R., Soltero, I., Stamler, R., Gosch, F., Stevens, E. and Stamler, J. (1979) Assessment of the association between habitual salt intake and high blood pressure: methodological problems. *American Journal of Epidemiology,* 11, 219.

Londe, S., Bourgoignie, J. J., Robson, A. M. and Goldring, D. (1971) Hypertension in apparently normal children. *Journal of Paediactrics,* 78, 569.

Lowenstein, F. W. (1961) Blood pressure in relation to age and sex in the tropics and sub-tropics. A review of the literature and an investigation in two tribes of Brazil Indians. *Lancet,* i, 389.

Maddocks, I. (1967) Blood pressure in Melanesians. *Medical Journal of Australia,* 1, 1123.

Malhotra, S. L. (1970) Dietary factors causing hypertension in India. *American Journal of Clinical Nutrition,* 23, 1353.

Malinow, M.R. (1980) Atherosclerosis. Regression in non-human primates. *Circulation Research,* 46, 311.

Marmot, M. G., Syme, S. L., Kagan, A., Kato, H., Cohen, J. B. and Belsky, J.

(1975) Epidemiologic studies of coronary heart disease and stroke in Japanese men living in Japan, Hawaii and California: prevalence of coronary and hypertensive heart disease and associated risk factors. *American Journal of Epidemiology,* **102,** 514.

Maxfield, E. and Konishi, F. (1966) Patterns of food intake and physical activity in obesity. *Journal of the American Dietetic Association,* **49,** 406.

McCance, R. A. and Widdowson, E. M. (1956) "Breads White and Brown". Pitman Medical Publishing, London.

McCarthy, M. C. (1966) Dietary and activity patterns of obese women in Trinidad. *Journal of the American Dietectic Association,* **48,** 33.

McGill, H. C. Jr (1968) "The Geographic Pathology of Atherosclerosis". Williams and Wilkins, Baltimore.

McGill, H. C. Jr (1974) The lesion. *In* "Atherosclerosis III", Proceedings of the Third International Symposium, G. Schettler, and A. Weizel, (eds). Springer Verlag, Berlin, Heidelberg and New York.

Meneely, G. R. and Batterbee, H. D. (1976) High sodium, low potassium environment and hypertension. *American Journal of Cardiology,* **38,** 768.

Meneely, G. R., Ball, C. O. T. and Youmans, J. B. (1957) Chronic sodium toxicity: the protective effect of added potassium chloride. *Annals of Internal Medicine,* **47,** 263.

Miall, W. E. and Oldham, P. D. (1963) The hereditary factor in arterial blood pressure. *British Medical Journal,* **1,** 75.

Miall, W. E., Heneage, P., Khosla, T., Lovell, H. S. and Moore, F. (1967) Factors influencing the degree of resemblance in arterial pressure of close relatives. *Clinical Science,* **33,** 271.

Miller, D. S. and Parsonage, S. (1975) Resistance to slimming: adaptation or illusion? *Lancet,* **i,** 773.

Miller, N. E., Thelle, D. S., Førde, O. H. and Mjøs, O. D. (1977) The Tromso Heart Study. High density lipoprotein and coronary heart disease: a prospective case-control study. *Lancet,* **i,** 965.

National Food Survey Committee, Household Food Consumption and Expenditure. Annual Reports. HMSO, London.

Nichaman, M. Z., Hamilton, H. B. Kagan, A., Grier, T., Sacks, S. T. and Syme, S. L. (1975) Epidemiologic studies of coronary heart disease and stroke in Japanese men living in Japan, Hawaii, and California: distribution of biochemical risk factors. *American Journal of Epidemiology,* **102,** 6, 491.

Nupuf, M. S. and Sutherland, W. H. F. (1979) High density lipoprotein levels in children of young men with ischaemic heart disease. *Atherosclerosis,* **33,** 365.

Nye, L. J. (1937) Blood pressure in the Australian Aboriginal with a consideration of possible aetiological factors in hyperpiesia and its relation to civilization. *Medical Journal of Australia,* **ii,** 1000.

Office of Population Censuses and Surveys. Mortality data by region (1969–73). Personal Communication.

Office of Population Censuses and Surveys (1977) Mortality statistics. HMSO, London.

Office of Population Censuses and Surveys (1978) Occupational Mortality. Dicennial Supplement 1970–72. HMSO, London.

Page, L. B., Danion, A. and Moellering, R. C. Jr (1974) Antecedents of cardiovascular disease in six Soloman Island societies. *Circulation,* **49,** 1132.

Paterson, D. and Slack, J. (1972) Lipid abnormalities in male and female survivors of myocardial infarction and their first degree relatives. *Lancet,* **i,** 393.

Pietinen, P. I., Wong, O. and Altschul, A. M. (1979) Electrolyte output, blood pressure and family history of hypertension. *American Journal of Clinical Nutrition,* **32,** 997.

Pooling Project Research Group (1978) Relationship of blood pressure, serum cholesterol, smoking habit, relative weight and E.C.G. abnormalities to incidence of major coronary events. Final report of the Pooling Project. *Journal of Chronic Diseases,* **31,** 201.

Prior, A. M., Evans, J. G., Harvey, H. P. B., Davidson, F. and Lindsey, M. (1968) Sodium intake and blood pressure in two Polynesian populations. *New England Journal of Medicine,* **279,** 515.

Renaud, J., Dumont, E, Godsey, F., Suplissaen, A. and Thevenon, C. (1979) Platelet functions in relation to dietary fats in farmers from two regions of France. *Thrombosis and Haemostasis,* **40,** 518.

Report from the International Agency for Research on Cancer Intestinal Microecology Group. (1977) Dietary fibre, transit-time, faecal bacteria, steroids and colon cancer in two Scandinavian populations. *Lancet,* **ii,** 207.

Robson, J. R. K., Bazin, M. and Soderstrom, R. (1971) Ethnic differences in skinfold thickness. *American Journal of Clinical Nutrition,* **24,** 864.

Rose, G. (1964) Familial patterns in ischaemic heart disease. *British Journal of Preventative and Social Medicine,* **18,** 75.

Rose, G. A. and Williams, T. R. (1961) Metabolic studies on large and small eaters. *British Journal of Nutrition,* **15,** 1.

Royal College of Physicians (1980) "Report on Medical Aspects of Dietary Fibre". Pitman Medical, London.

Sasaki, N. (1962) High blood pressure and the salt intake of the Japanese. *Japan Heart Journal,* **3,** 313.

Sasaki, N. (1964) The relationship of salt intake to hypertension in the Japanese. *Geriatrics,* **19,** 735.

Sasaki, N., Mitsuhasi, T. and Fukushi, S. (1959) Effects of the ingestion of large amounts of apples on blood pressure in farmers in Akitu prefectures. *Igaku to Seibutsugaka,* **51,** 103.

Saunders, G. M. (1932) Blood pressure in Yucatecans. *American Journal of Medical Science,* **185,** 843.

Schroeder, H. A. (1958) Degenerative cardiovascular disease in the Orient. II. Hypertension. *Journal of Chronic Diseases,* **8,** 312.

Shaper, A. G. (1962) Cardiovascular studies in the Samburu tribe of Northern Kenya. *American Heart Journal,* **63,** 437.

Shaper, A. G. (1972) Cardiovascular disease in the tropics. IV. Coronary artery disease. *British Medical Journal,* **4,** 32.

Shaper, A. G., Leonard, P. J., Jones, K. W. and Jones, M. (1969) Environmental effects on the body build, blood pressure and blood chemistry of nomadic warriors serving in the army in Kenya. *East African Medical Journal,* **46,** 282.

Sharrett, A. R. and Feinleib, M. (1975) Water constituents and trace elements in relation to cardiovascular disease. *Preventative Medicine,* **4,** 20.

Shetty, P. S., Jung, R. T., James, W. P. T., Barrand, M. A. and Callingham, B. A. (1981) Postprandial thermogenesis in obesity. *Clinical Science* (in press).

Sims, E. A. H., Danforth, E., Horton, E. S., Bray, G. A., Glennow, J. A. and Salams, L. B. (1973) Endocrine and metabolic effects of experimental obesity in man. *Recent Progress in Hormone Research,* **29,** 457.

Slack, J. (1969) Risks of ischaemic heart disease in familial hyperlipoproteinaemic states. *Lancet,* **ii,** 1380.

Slack, J. (1975) The genetic contribution to coronary heart disease through lipoprotein concentrations. *Postgraduate Medical Journal,* **51** (Suppl. 8), 27.

Southgate, D. A. T., Bingham, S. and Robertson, J. (1978) Dietary Fibre in the British Diet. *Nature,* **274,** 51.

Srinivasan, S. R., Berenson, G. S., Radhakrishnamusthy, B., Dalferes, E. R., Underwood, D. and Foster, T. A. (1980) Effects of dietary sodium and sucrose on the induction of hypertension in Spider monkeys. *American Journal of Clinical Nutrition,* **33,** 561.

Sveger, T., Lindberg, T., Weibull, B. and Olssen, U. L. (1975) Nutrition, over-nutrition and obesity in the first year of life in Malmö, Sweden. *Acta Paediatrica Scandinavica,* **64,** 635.

Takahashi, E. (1978) *In* "Ecologic Human Biology in Japan", p. 129. Medical Information Services.

Thurlby, P. L. and Trayhurn, P. (1980) Regional blood flow in genetically obese (ob/ob) mice: the importance of brown adipose tissue to the reduced energy expenditure on non-shivering thermogenesis. *Pflugers Archiv für die gesamte Physiologie des Menschen und der Tiere,* **385,** 193.

Trenchard, Rt Hon. Viscount (1977) Fat Consumption Assumptions. *Meat Trades Journal,* Sept. 29, 4–5.

Truswell, A. S. (1977) Diet and nutrition of hunter gatherers. Ciba Foundation Symposium 49 (New Series), p. 213.

Tung, C. L. (1927) Relative hypotension of foreigners in China. *Archives of Internal Medicine,* **40,** 153.

Van der Haar, F. and Kromhout, D. (1978) Food intake, nutritional anthropometry and blood chemical parameters in 3 selected Dutch schoolchildren populations. Communications, Agricultural University, Wageningen, The Netherlands, No. 78–9.

Vaughan, J. P. and Miall, W. E. (1979) A comparison of cardiovascular measurements in the Gambia, Jamaica and the United Republic of Tanzania. *Bulletin of the World Health Organization,* **57,** 281.

Vesselinovitch, D., Wissler, R. W., Schaffner, T. J. and Borensztajn, J. (1980) The effect of various diets on atherogenesis in rhesus monkeys. *Atherosclerosis,* **35,** 189.

Veterans Administration Co-operative Study Group on Antihypertensive Agents (1967) Effects of treatment on morbidity in hypertension. Results in patients with diastolic blood pressure averaging 115 through 129 mmHg. *Journal of the American Medical Association,* **202,** 1028.

Veterans Administration Co-operative Study Group on Hypertensive Agents (1970) Effects of treatment on morbidity in hypertension. II. Results in patients with diastolic blood pressure averaging 90 through 114 mmHg. *Journal of the American Medical Association* **213,** 1143.

Vlodaver, Z., Kahn, H. A. and Neufeld, H. N. (1969) The coronary arteries in early life in three different ethnic groups. *Circulation,* **31,** 541.

Vobecky, J., Vobecky, J. S., Shapcott, D., Demers, P.-P., Reid, D., Fisch, C., Blanchard, R., Cloutier, D. and Black, R. (1979) Food intake patterns of infants with high serum cholesterol level at six months. *International Journal of Vitamin and Nutrition Research,* **49,** 189.

Weidman, W. H., Eloeback, L. R., Nelson, R. A., Hodgson, P. A. and Ellefson, R. D. (1978) Nutrient intake and serum cholesterol level in normal children 6 to 16 years of age. *Pediatrics,* **61,** 354.

Whyte, H. M. (1958) Body fat and blood pressure of natives in New Guinea: reflections on essential hypertension. *Australian Annals of Medicine,* **7,** 36.

Widdowson, E. M. (1962) Nutritional individuality. *Proceedings of the Nutritional Society,* **21,** 121.

Wiggins, R. C., Basar, I. and Slater, J. D. H. (1978) Effect of arterial pressure and inheritance on the sodium excretory capacity of normal young men. *Clinical Science and Molecular Medicine* **54,** 639.

Wilens, S. L. (1951) The nature of diffuse intimal thickening of arteries. *American Journal of Pathology,* **27,** 825.

Williams, D. R. R. (1980) Salt intake and the pathenogenesis of hypertension: population studies. Nutritional Bulletin 28, vol. 5, no. 4, pp. 187–93.

World Health Statistics Annual (1979) 3 vols. World Health Organization, Geneva.

Worth, R. M., Kato, H., Rhoads, G. G., Kagan, A. and Syme, S. L. (1975) Epidemiological studies of coronary heart disease and stroke in Japanese men living in Japan, Hawaii and California: Mortality. *American Journal of Epidemiology,* **102,** 481.

Young, J. B. and Landsberg, L. (1978) Fasting, feeding and regulation of the sympathetic nervous system. *New England Journal of Medicine,* **298,** 1295.

The Cost of Diet-related Diseases

W. A. Laing

Office of Health Economics, London

The primary objective of this paper is to provide estimates of the costs to society of those diseases which are known, or believed, to have major dietary components. The data are set out in an Appendix, following the principles generally accepted by economists specializing in health services.

Some of these costs, in particular the ones borne by the National Health Service (NHS), can be estimated with reasonable confidence. By that I mean that relative errors are unlikely to be in excess of 20%. In other cases NA, meaning "not available", has been entered in appropriate columns of the Appendix to signify that, although there is no satisfactory basis for estimating their magnitude, real costs nevertheless exist.

The paper will then address itself to those issues which bear upon the values of preventive intervention. It will come as no surprise that precise calculations of the anticipated costs and benefits of any given preventive measure cannot be offered. There are three basic reasons why. First there is a lack of data required to predict, quantitatively, change in health status resulting from a given dietary change. Second, there is a similar lack of data required to predict, quantitatively, the dietary change resulting from a given form of intervention. (N.B. these two are largely the province of epidemiologists.) Third, there is an absence of any agreed convention on (or even any agreed approach to) what comparative values to place on different health care "outputs"; in particular, how to value changes in "health status" on the same scale as changes in "resources". (N.B. This is largely the province of economists.)

This emphasis on the problems of measurement should not be interpreted as suggesting that analysis is of little value. Rather, I want to put over the point that a *finely tuned* model for producing cost/benefit "results" across the range of health issues is not a practicable proposition and will not be for a long time to come, if ever. A growing body of opinion is accepting more limited and more realistic objectives of analysis, namely: of informing public debate within a logical analytical framework; of exposing the value judgements that lie behind particular methods of analysis; and of highlighting the orders of magnitude of costs and benefits. Occasionally, the magnitudes will be such that, even though approximate, the implications for public policy will be obvious.

Finally, an illustration will be given of the potential benefits of the prevention of certain diseases by dietary change.

Estimation of costs

In the Appendix the costs of diseases are divided into two classes. The first is headed "resources". The figures entered under here represent estimates of the impact of each disease on the resources available to the community. These include the "direct" costs of health services and the so-called "indirect" costs of loss of productive potential through sickness and premature death. The second class is "health status".

Health status

The figures which should ideally appear under the heading of health status would represent money values of the loss of well-being or loss of life resulting from each disease. That is, they would represent personal losses to individuals *as individuals,* rather than to individuals *as factors of production.* These costs have often been called "intangibles". The word "intangible" is, however, inappropriate. The changes in health status which it is intended to describe are very real, representing as they do the realization of the primary purpose of health services. Nevertheless, no one has yet found a sound basis for translating them into money terms, so NA (not available) has been entered against the personal cost of pain, disability and distress to patients and their families. The number of deaths in a year has been entered as a quantitative proxy for one aspect of the burden of disease on individuals.

Resource costs

It is necessary to consider in some detail the methods used to estimate the resource costs of diseases and to discuss the assumptions upon which they are based and the likely magnitudes of error.

Direct costs

Direct costs are almost wholly composed of NHS costs. The same basic method was used throughout. That is, the total cost of each sector, shown

Table I

Estimated NHS revenue[a] expenditure in the UK in
1979/80 (Office of Health Economics estimates from
various sources).

	£ million
Hospital revenue[a] expenditure	
In-patients in non-psychiatric hospitals and units	3746
In-patients in mental illness and mental handicap hospitals and units	873
Out-patients	589
Accident and emergency, day patients, day cases and other patients (no basis for allocating expenditure by disease)	344
	5552
Other revenue[a] expenditure	
Community health services	627
Pharmaceutical services[b]	1077
General medical services	572
Dental services[b]	386
Ophthalmic services[b]	47
TOTAL REVENUE EXPENDITURE	8261

[a]Capital expenditure, central administration and certain
miscellaneous, centrally funded items are excluded from
the table.
[b]Figures are gross of NHS charges but net of expenditure on
private services.

in Table I, was apportioned between diseases by the use of such measures of
resource usage that were available from public or private sources.
International Classification of Diseases (ICD) categories were used
throughout. Thus any possibility of overlap was avoided and summation
for all conditions, whether diet-related or not, would give totals equal to the
overall cost of each sector considered.

In one instance, the cost of over-the-counter medicines was available but
generally these have been excluded from the analysis. The private medical
sector has been excluded entirely; at present this accounts for between 1 and
2% of health care spending in the UK. More important, other direct costs
such as local authority care for disabled people have had to be excluded
because there is no basis for apportionment by disease. Finally, within the
estimated net revenue expenditure of £8261 million on the NHS in the UK in

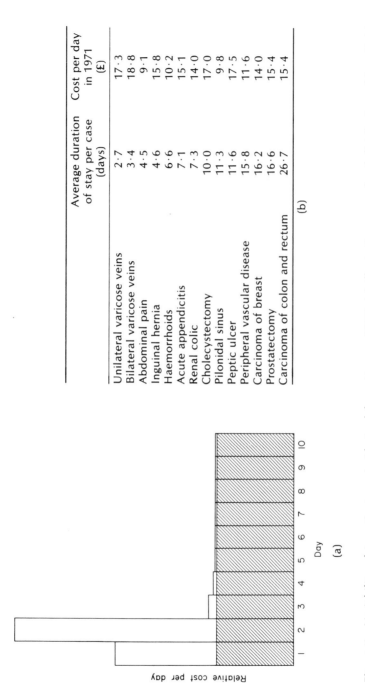

	Average duration of stay per case (days)	Cost per day in 1971 (£)
Unilateral varicose veins	2·7	17·3
Bilateral varicose veins	3·4	18·8
Abdominal pain	4·5	9·1
Inguinal hernia	4·6	15·8
Haemorrhoids	6·6	10·2
Acute appendicitis	7·1	15·1
Renal colic	7·3	14·0
Cholecystectomy	10·0	17·0
Pilonidal sinus	11·3	9·8
Peptic ulcer	11·6	17·5
Peripheral vascular disease	15·8	11·6
Carcinoma of breast	16·2	14·0
Prostatectomy	16·6	15·4
Carcinoma of colon and rectum	26·7	15·4

(b)

Figure 1 Variability of in-patients costs (derived from Harper, 1979). (a) Illustrative example of distribution of hospital in-patient costs by day of stay. Unshaded areas represent direct costs, e.g. drugs, nursing time, medical time, generated directly by patients care. Shaded areas represent "overheads", e.g. catering and laundry, largely independent of case mix, and apportioned per patient bed-day (derived from Babson, 1973). (b) Variation in in-patient costs by selected condition (derived from Harper, 1979).

1979/80 (Table I), £344 million—representing expenditure on accident and emergency services, day patients, day cases and other patients—could not be allocated by disease. To reflect the fact that such other costs exist but cannot be estimated, a column headed "other direct costs" has been included in the Appendix and "NA" entered against each condition.

Hospital in-patient costs   Hospital in-patient costs comprise by far the largest cost sector. For non-psychiatric hospitals and units the basis of apportionment was bed occupancy taken from the latest (1975) hospital in-patient enquiry (DHSS/OPCS/Welsh Office, 1979). The data are generated from a 10% sample of patients. For psychatric hospitals and units (only relevant for alcoholism) the 1976 census of patients was used (DHSS, 1979). For a number of conditions bed occupancy data were not available at a sufficiently detailed level of disaggregation. In these cases discharges and deaths were used as a basis for apportionment and this is indicated, where appropriate, in the Appendix.

The major source of error in these calculations lies in the implicitly assumed homogeneity of bed occupancy in terms of costs. That is, it is assumed that one bed-day for the diagnosis "stomach cancer" costs the same as a bed-day for the diagnosis "ischaemic heart disease". Perhaps more important, it assumes that cost per bed-day does not vary with duration of stay.

However, what few data exist do not give a consistent picture of the size or even the direction of likely errors. Figure 1 illustrates the point. Here, Babson's data (1973) reflect what is well known, namely that most of the variable costs occur in the first few days of hospitalization. It might be concluded, therefore, that the methods outlined above will underestimate the cost of those conditions where duration of stay is short and over-estimate for those where it is long. On the other hand Harper's data (1979), collected over a six-month period in a surgical ward, show no relationship between duration of stay and cost per day for the different types of case he considered.

The standard deviation of costs per day for the surgical conditions considered by Harper, expressed as a proportion of the mean of costs per day, is 20%. In the absence of anything more satisfactory this can be used as a very rough indication of the order of magnitude of error that might arise from assumed homogeneity of costs in the data in the Appendix.

Where discharges have been used to estimate bed occupancy a further source of significant error arises from assumed equivalence of duration of stay between conditions.

Out-patient costs   The basis of apportionment of out-patient costs is the Second National Morbidity Study of 1971/2 (Royal College of General Practioners/OPCS/DHSS, 1979). Table 14 of that publication lists out-patient referrals by disease. The major sources of error are probably the age of the data; the composition of the (self selected) general practitioners in the sample of 43 practices; and the implicit assumption that referrals to out-patient resource use by disease.

Cost of domiciliary services   Included in the category of domiciliary services are general medical services, the pharmaceutical service and general dental services.

Data for apportionment of the cost of the first two sectors are taken from the Medical Data Index for 1978, made available by IMS Ltd, a market research organization which regularly collects information from a rotating sample of 200 general practitioners. General medical services have been apportioned on the basis of numbers of consultations by diagnosis and pharmaceutical services on the basis of prescription numbers by diagnosis. The major sources of error are the assumptions that consultations for each disease consume equivalent resources (GP time) and that the cost per prescription is equivalent for each disease. These assumptions are clearly invalid but the Medical Data Index data provide, nevertheless, better approximations than those of the Second National Morbidity Study of which Table B (consultations by diagnosis) have been used as a measure of resource use in previous publications (Black and Pole, 1975). The advantages of the IMS data are: they are more recent; the sample of GPs is closer to a random sample of all GPs in Britain; there is a direct measure of prescription numbers as well as consultations by disease.

Indirect costs

The so-called indirect costs of diseases raise difficult conceptual problems. I shall look first of all at "production lost due to sickness absence". It is worth considering the problems in some detail since the figures are so large.

A reasonable starting position is that when an employee goes off sick the work that is not done has the approximate value of his or her salary. Therefore, multiplying days of absence recorded by the DHSS (for which sickness or invalidity benefit was claimed) by the average income per day for males and for females gives an estimate of "lost production".

This is a procedure which has often been used in the past. However, it may be argued that this overestimates the real loss of production in that an increase of sickness absence at the margin results in an induced inflow of people from the pool of unemployed into employment. To this extent the opportunity cost of marginal days of sickness absence (i.e. the production lost) is zero.

In principle, therefore, it is necessary to reduce estimates of production lost due to sickness absence by an amount obtained by integrating the function: change in unemployment over change in days of sickness absence—over a given range of sickness absence levels, i.e.

$$\text{Income per day} \quad \times \quad \begin{array}{l} \text{days of sickness absence} = \chi_1 \\ \text{days of sickness absence} = \chi_0 \end{array} \int f(\chi) \, d\chi,$$

where $f(\chi)$ is used to represent the rate of change of days of unemployment with respect to days of sickness absence over a given range.[1]

I have no idea what a graph of $f(\chi)$ would look like, except that its magnitude would presumably be a monotonically increasing function of unemployment levels.

There is yet another conceptual problem which is particularly important when considering potential savings from dietary change. It is well recognized that short-term sickness absence is a social rather than a medical phenomenon (Office of Health Economics, 1971). Researchers usually refer to "absence *attributed* to sickness" as a means of emphasizing that diseases are very often a convenient label for legitimizing a decision to stay off work for other reasons. Thus a given reduction in the incidence of a diet-related disease would certainly not give rise to a corresponding reduction in sickness absence.

Each of these points suggests the real cost of sickness absence is overestimated in the Appendix. For the sake of completeness, it should be mentioned that there are sources of considerable underestimation as well. DHSS data on absence exclude absence of uninsured employed people such as married women. They also exclude incapacity amongst non-employed disabled people and amongst housewives whose work, though lacking a market price, must be accounted for in a fully comprehensive analysis.

Clearly, "lost production" figures are to be treated with some caution. The same may be said of the other category of indirect cost, lost production due to premature mortality. In early publications it was the established convention to value lost life years at the gross income of the individual, as a measure of his/her production. A later refinement was to reduce this by the individual's expected consumption.

Because of unresolved conceptual and accounting difficulties I have made no attempt to place values on the change of resources available to the community as a consequence of deaths from diet-related diseases. Once again, however, it is important to recognize that real changes of wealth would arise from the prevention of mortality. It is also important to

---

[1]It might also be argued that to some extent sickness absence represents a voluntary redistribution of working and leisure time and that one of the effects of a general reduction in sickness absence levels may be pressure towards a reduction in the formal length of the working week. To that extent any estimated "gains" would be illusory.

recognize that such changes in wealth would not necessarily be beneficial. To the extent that preventive measures extend the lives of *non-employed* people there must be a *debit* entry under "resources" in the balance sheet. This would of course be separate from the (unknown) value of life *per se* to individuals and their families and friends.

In order to give some quantitative indication of the resource consequences of preventable mortality I have calculated "life years lost" by multiplying the number of deaths (in the UK in 1977) in each age and sex group by expectation of life from English Life tables. The resulting "life years lost" have been divided into those under 65 and those over 65 as an approximation to employed and non-employed life years. In almost every case it may be noted, non-employed life-years exceed employed life years.

Transfer payments

The final column in the Appendix is "Sickness and invalidity benefits: transfers from government to individuals". I have separated this column from the others because it represents neither a health status item nor a resource item but rather a redistribution or purchasing power from government to individuals. The magnitude of these transfers is naturally a matter of concern for society but conceptually the *resource* cost of sickness absence has already been counted under "Production lost".

Cost effectiveness of prevention by dietary change

Having estimated, albeit incompletely, the burden of diet-related diseases it remains to ask to what extent preventive measures are worthwhile. It is at this stage that one becomes acutely aware of the paucity of data with which to fill in any conceptual framework, whether simple or sophisticated, for assessing benefits in relation to costs. The data requirements can be illustrated as in Fig. 2.

Valuation of health

It would be inappropriate to spend a great deal of time discussing the often intricate and obscure controversies surrounding the valuation of health outputs. In summary, however, no consensus has yet developed on how to

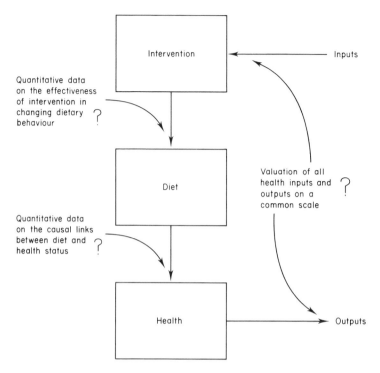

Figure 2 Diagrammatic illustration of data requirements for comprehensive analysis of the costs and benefits of preventive intervention.

quantify the subjective value of being alive and healthy to individuals themselves. All that can be said is that, ideally, a procedure is required which would allow all costs and benefits to be set against each other in common terms, such as money. It may be that such an objective is impossible. In that case, it would be necessary for the idealized policy maker to place his own subjective valuations on each class of cost or benefit flowing from a given form of intervention.

Epidemiological data

In recent years a good deal of epidemiological data has become available demonstrating the link between diet and major diseases. But, understandably, most studies have been primarily concerned with establishing the existence of casual links and with meeting tests of statistical significance. They rarely generate the sort of data that might form the basis for calculating, even approximately, the risks of excess morbidity/mortality attributable to incremental increases in the dietary factors concerned and thus for estimating the potential benefit from preventive intervention.

The Finnish mental hospitals study (Turpeinen, 1979) is exceptional in this respect. It was an attempt to measure, in a controlled experiment, the effect of replacing a "normal" diet with a "serum cholesterol lowering" diet in which "soft margarine" and "filled milk" replaced butter and milk. Some of its results can be used to illustrate how the requirements for calculating precise costs and benefits are very unlikely ever to be met (Fig. 3).

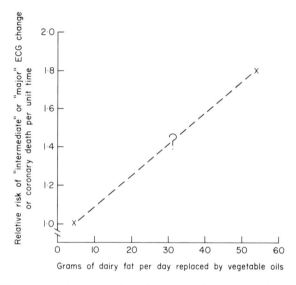

Figure 3   Illustration of potential benefit from replacing dairy fat with vegetable oils using data from the Finnish Mental Hospitals study (op. cit.). (Risk of morbidity/mortality from "serum cholesterol lowering" diet = 1.)

Leaving aside questions of validity of the study, the economist or planner wishing to estimate potential benefits from prevention has the following problems:

1) It may not be justifiable to extrapolate results to populations which are genetically, environmentally or culturally different.

2) Only two points are shown on the graph and it may not be justifiable to interpolate between them to estimate incremental changes in morbidity and mortality over the entire range of fat intake.

3) The results say nothing about age differences in response or about time lags between intervention and response.

4) The morbidity data are unlikely to be recorded in a manner which a cost/benefit analyst would choose.

It is highly unlikely that sufficient long-term controlled trials could be done in the foreseeable future to meet the exacting requirements implicit in the comments above.

For other diet-related diseases, e.g. dental caries, a more highly developed theory of the causal link between the main dietary factor (sugar) and the condition, may facilitate analysis. Thus Best (1979) has suggested that for every additional ton of sugar-containing foodstuffs consumed in the UK there will be a need for more than 50 courses of dental treatment. Here as well, however, empirical data fall far short of what is required for a precise and comprehensive analysis of the costs and benefits of restricting sugar consumption.

To expect a high degree of precision in cost/benefit analysis is therefore futile. Approximations with wide error bounds and entire blank areas will have to be accepted for the foreseeable future.

The relationship between intervention and dietary change

Research focusing on the effectiveness of nutritional intervention *per se* is in its infancy (Tolpin, 1980). What quantitative data are available can at best give only very approximate ideas of the likely impact of preventive intervention. Nevertheless, there is evidence that the dietary behaviour of communities can be changed. For example, in North Karelia in Finland, it was found that serum cholesterol levels were reduced significantly compared with a control community following a comprehensive five-year community programme to control cardiovascular diseases.

Forms of preventive intervention

There are a number of different forms that preventive intervention may take, each of which would have its own cost profile and set of special considerations.

On the one hand a programme of health education may be aimed at a particular community with the objective of altering behaviour in specific ways. Examples include the North Karelia project. Also included would be less comprehensive campaigns such as those financed, for example, by the

Health Education Council in Britain. Given the wide range of behaviour which educational campaigns have attempted to modify it is not surprising that few generalizations can be made, except that results are often disappointing and it is easy to waste money on programmes which have no theoretical basis derived from research findings.

An alternative approach may be to aim at key stages of opinion and behaviour formation. Thus nutritional education in schools may be more cost effective than campaigns conducted through the mass media. Clearly there is a need for more research of a high standard in this whole area in order better to inform policy makers. On the positive side it may be noted that mortality from cardiovascular diseases has shown a marked decline in the USA and other industrialized countries. Some of this decline may be attributable to dietary change and clearly a climate of opinion has developed in which behaviour may be modified.

Intervention could also take place at the level of the food producer, perhaps through legislation. In this case extra costs may be involved in manufacturing processes, costs which must be taken into account together with health consequences, in any comprehensive analysis of costs and benefits. It may be argued that, theoretically and in the long term, resources used in the production of one kind of food could be reallocated to produce another kind of food. But it would be naive to suppose that change would not be opposed on account of the dislocation and the effect on commercial and national financial interests that would result. At this level dietary prevention becomes frankly political and the lack of energy with which governments have in the past pursued health objectives in opposition to economic interests (e.g. smoking and drinking) is not encouraging.

Potential benefits from prevention of diet-related diseases

There are few conditions which could not in some way be associated with diet. Thus data from the Metropolitan Life Insurance Company in the USA show excess mortality from many diseases amongst overweight people. In the Appendix I have, I think, included every ICD category for which there is reasonable scientific evidence for a link between some dietary factor and incidence. In Table II the analysis is taken a stage further by estimating, for certain selected conditions on which good evidence of causal links exists, the "dietary component". This is intended to represent the approximate proportion of cases that might potentially be prevented by dietary change under the particular genetic and environmental conditions of Britain in the 1980s, regardless of whether or not the conditions could be prevented by other additional environmental change.

Clearly, the proportions must be taken as illustrative only. The "dietary components" are in some cases higher than those assumed in a similar illustrative exercise undertaken with Canadian data (Sabry, 1975). On the other hand, the diagnostic categories I have used are more specific. It may be argued that a number of conditions on which there is adequate evidence of a dietary factor in the causation have not been included in Table II. In those cases "potential benefits" can be generated in a similar way by applying whatever "dietary component" is felt appropriate to the data in the Appendix. It is because it is unlikely that there will be agreement on exactly which illnesses should appear that I make no attempt to estimate the "total" burden of diet-related diseases.

In terms of direct health-care costs the two most important conditions in Table II are diseases of the hard tissues of the teeth and ischaemic heart disease. For diseases of the teeth it is assumed that 75% of the cost to the NHS (almost all accounted for by the dental service) could be saved by a reduction in dental caries following the total elimination of sweet and sticky food and drinks from the British diet. However, it is unrealistic to assume that this would be possible. In any case, the *consequences* of changes in consumption of sweet foods are not as straightforward in economic terms. Careful consideration of the case justifies the emphasis placed on the need to develop a comprehensive framework for analysis, even if there are considerable gaps in data. For example, if incidence of dental caries were so high as to lead to provision of dentures at an early age for a large proportion of the population, that may turn out cheaper in NHS resources than long-term conservation given a moderate incidence of caries. To gain some idea of costs and benefits it is necessary to be aware of the magnitude of *all* the resource consequences of a given policy and the trade-offs between these and the health status consequences, in this case the utility derived from having one's own teeth.

Ischaemic heart disease further illustrates the importance of a comprehensive framework for analysis. In this case there is a theoretical benefit of some £100 million in NHS resource savings, but the net value of preventive intervention will depend critically on the unestimated, but undoubtedly much larger, magnitude of production lost through sickness absence (potential gain), productive life years lost through premature death (potential gain) and non-productive life years (potential loss).

Table II

Annual potential benefits from changes in dietary habits (1979/80 prices) in the UK for certain selected conditions.

Condition	Dietary factor	Dietary component	Resources		Health status	Other quantitative indicators; deaths preventible and life-years savable		
			Direct NHS costs preventible per year (£ million)	Other direct costs and indirect costs preventible per year (£ million)	Total personal distress preventible (£ million)	Deaths 1975 (England and Wales)	Life years[a] (from 1975 data) Under 65	65 and over
Constipation[b] ICD 564·0	Dietary fibre	100	26	NA	NA	15	6	146
Diverticula of the intestine ICD 562	Dietary fibre	100	10	NA	NA	1376	1450	12,821
Diabetes mellitus	obesity (mature onset diabetes)	80	67	NA	NA	3911	1125	39,990
Alcoholism ICD 303 and cirrhosis of the liver ICD 571	Alcohol	100	76[c]	NA	NA	609[d]	8303[d]	7408[d]

Obesity not specified as of endocrine origin ICD 277	Obesity	100	14	NA	NA	177	1222	2159
Cancer of the large intestine ICD 153	Dietary fibre	100	28	NA	NA	10,346	26,969	109,217
Cholelithiasis ICD 574		100	25	NA	NA	524	765	4716
Ischaemic heart disease ICD 410–414	Animal fat	50	97	NA	NA	77,906	169,690	752,984
Diseases of the hard tissues of the teeth ICD 521	Sweet and sticky food and drinks	70	271	NA	NA	0	0	0

[a]Life years "saved" in a given year include all future "expected" life years according to English life tables. Thus similar calculations relating to subsequent years would have to be adjusted to avoid double counting.

[b]Including £7·1 million of hospital in-patient costs attributable to "functional disorders of the intestines" ICD 564. Out-patient costs not estimated owing to lack of data.

[c]Composed of £72·0 million for Alcoholism, ICD 303 and £3·5 million for cirrhosis of the liver, ICD 571.

[d]Deaths and life years attributable to alcoholic cirrhosis, ICD 571·0.

Conclusions

The data in Table II show that there are potential benefits of a very large order of magnitude from the prevention of diet-related diseases. It is, therefore, clearly worth giving a very high priority to dietary change and to high quality research into means of achieving such changes. At the very least, the return from even marginally effective preventive intervention is likely to be significantly greater than the return from curative intervention which at present consumes nearly all the resources of the NHS.

THE PRACTICAL QUESTION IS, WHAT LEVEL OF CERTAINTY AS TO OUTCOME IS REQUIRED BEFORE A DECISION TO COMMIT RESOURCES SHOULD BE MADE? At one end of the continuum the intellectually unassailable position might be taken that hard data from controlled trials of a particular form of intervention should be the prerequisite of policy change. On the other hand, a less demanding position may be appropriate. That is, if there are very large benefits to be gained and a reasonable expectation, on the balance of evidence, that intervention will be effective to some degree, then that may be sufficient for committing resources. This sort of question is likely to be increasingly debated.

References

Babson, J. H. (1973) "Disease Costing. Studies in Social Administration". Manchester University Press.

Best, G. A. (1979) "Notes on the macroeconomics of illness and health". Discussion Paper No. 67, Department of Economics, Birkbeck College, London.

Black, D. and Pole, J. (1975) Priorities in biomedical research. Indices of burden. *British Journal of Preventative and Social Medicine*, **29**, 222–27.

Department of Health and Social Security OPCS Welsh Office (1979) "Hospital In Patient Enquiry. England and Wales". HMSO, London. Main tables 1975.

Department of Health and Social Security (1979) "In Patient Statistics from the Mental Health Enquiry for England 1976". Statistical and Research Report Series No. 22. HMSO, London.

Harper, D. R. (1979) Disease cost in a surgical ward. *British Medical Journal*, **1**, 647–9.

Office of Health Economics (1971) "Off Sick". OHE, London.

Royal College of General Practitioners OPCS Department of Health and Social Security (1979). "Morbidity Statistics from General Practice. Second National Study". Studies on Medical and Population Subjects No. 36. HMSO, London.

Sabry, Z. I. (1975) The cost of malnutrition in Canada. *Canadian Journal of Public Health*, **66**, 291–3.

Tolpin, H. G. (1980) Economics of health care. *Journal of the American Dietetic Association*, **76**, 217–22.

Turpeinen, O. (1979) Dietary prevention of coronary heart disease. *International Journal of Epidemiology*, **8**, 99–118.

Appendix

Annual costs of diseases in the United Kingdom, 1979/80, prices.

Disease	Resources				Indirect costs			Health status		
	Direct costs					"Production lost" through premature death. Measured as years of life lost under and over age 65 (1975 mortality rate)				
	Hospital in-patient costs	Hospital out-patient costs	Domiciliary costs (GPs, prescription medicines, dentists)	Other direct costs	"Production lost" through sickness absence	Under 65	65 and over	Personal cost of pain, and distress to patients and their families	Deaths (England and Wales, 1975)	Sickness and invalidity benefit. Transfers from government to individuals
					(£ million)					
Food poisoning (bacterial) ICD 005	0·4[a]	NA	0	NA	NA	0	15	NA	2	NA
Stomach cancer ICD 151	16·7[a]	0·5	1·2	NA	2·2	25,585	117,424	NA	11,370	0·6[b]
Cancer of the large intestine ICD 153	27·1[a]	0·6	0·6	NA	2·4[b]	26,969	109,217	NA	10,346	0·7[b]
Breast cancer ICD 174	35·0	2·8	1·6	NA	1·7[b]	170,144	162,079	NA	11,918	0·7[b]
Diabetes mellitus ICD 250	63·2	4·0	16·2	NA	60·9	14,059	49,988	NA	4889	17·0

(cont.)

Avitaminoses and other nutritional deficiency ICD 260—269	12·5[a]	0·1	1·7	NA	1·6	375	46	NA	208	0·4
Obesity not specified as of endocrine origin ICD 277	3·0[a]	0·6	10·0	NA	26·8[b]	1222	2157	NA	177	8·1[b]
Iron deficiency anaemias ICD 280	6·9[a]	1·5	3·9	NA	10·6[b]	151	1107	NA	136	3·4[b]
Alcoholism ICD 303	69·9[a]	0·3	1·8	NA	NA	3374	2219	NA	181	NA
Malignant hypertension ICD 400	1·4[a]	NA	0·1	NA	NA	2251	2491	NA	200	NA
Essential benign hypertension ICD 401	17·2[a]	NA	83·4	NA	NA	1728	7413	NA	746	NA
Hypertensive heart disease ICD 402	3·5[a]	NA	4·7	NA	NA	8988	54,067	NA	5605	NA
Hypertensive renal disease ICD 403	0·8[a]	NA	0	NA	NA	1194	4855	NA	508	NA
Hypertensive heart and renal disease ICD 404	1·4[a]	NA	0	NA	NA	569	1593	NA	166	NA
Hypertensive disease ICD 400—404	23·1	5·2	82·7	NA	181·8	14,724	70,419	NA	7225	49·8

Acute myocardial infarction ICD 410	90·2	1·7	3·5	NA	129·3	NA	259,804	1,067,613	NA	105,712	34·3
Ischaemic heart disease ICD 410–414	154·7	5·3	34·7	NA	424·9	NA	339,380	1,505,967	NA	155,813	113·1
Cerebral haemorrhage ICD 431	19·3[a]	NA	0·1	NA	NA	NA	25,426	114,544	NA	11,634	NA
Generalized ischaemic cerebrovascular disease ICD 437	42·2[a]	NA	2·3	NA	NA	NA	1089	58,463	NA	8818	NA
Cerebrovascular disease ICD 430–438	358·3	2·4	6·8	NA	85·9	NA	93,302	639,858	NA	73,338	23·3
Arteriosclerosis ICD 440	19·1	NA	2·3	NA	NA	NA	1464	56,935	NA	9211	NA
Diseases of hard tissue of the teeth ICD 521	2·2[a]	NA	386·0	NA	10·6	NA	0	0	NA	0	3·2
Ulcer of the stomach and duodenum and peptic ulcer ICD 531–533	31·8	3·8	10·5	NA	65·7	NA	8655	38,998	NA	4134	17·6
Gastrojejunal ulcer ICD 535	0·4[a]	NA	0	NA	NA	NA	156	255	NA	29	NA

(cont.)

Appendix (cont.)

Gastritis and duodenitis ICD 535	2·1[a]	NA	9·7	NA	46·9	227	681	NA	76	13·3
Appendicitis ICD 540–543	34·9	1·1	0·2	NA	16·0	2325	2416	NA	229	4·7
Diverticula of the intestine ICD 562	8·0[a]	NA	2·2	NA	NA	1450	12,821	NA	1376	NA
Chronic enteritis and ulcerative colitis ICD 563	6·9[a]	NA	2·1	NA	NA	3414	4910	NA	440	NA
Cirrhosis of the liver ICD 571 (Deaths and life years represent alcoholic/ cirrhosis ICD 571·0)	3·4[a]	NA	0·1	NA	NA	4929	5189	NA	428	NA
Cholelithiasis ICD 574	24·4[a]	NA	0·6	NA	NA	765	4716	NA	524	NA
Constipation ICD 564·0	NA	NA	19·6[c]	NA	19·1[b]	6	146	NA	15	5·5[b]
Functional disorders of the intestines ICD 564	7·1[a]	NA	19·2	NA	NA	162	301	NA	32	NA
Anaemia of pregnancy ICD 633	0·5[a]	NA	0·3	NA	NA	0	0	NA	0	NA

Pre-eclampsia, eclampsia and toxaemia, unspecified ICD 637	5·3[a]	NA	0·1	NA	NA	389	114	NA	9	NA
Spontaneous abortion ICD 643	2·2[a]	NA	0·1	NA	NA	43	14	NA	1	NA
Rheumatoid arthritis and allied conditions ICD 712	56·2	3·3	13·0	NA	213·3	1947	10,722	NA	950	62·3
Osteo-arthritis and spondylitis ICD 713	68·2	9·5	43·6	NA	170·1	262	3232	NA	417	47·4
Arthritis and spondylitis ICD 710–715	138·0	NA	123·7	NA	NA	2993	15,632	NA	1926	NA
Certain causes of perinatal morbidity and mortality ICD 760–779	42·7	0	0·2	NA	0	238,485	28,994	NA	3356	0

[a]In-patient costs estimated from more highly aggregated disease classifications by assuming that bed occupancy is proportional to discharges and deaths within that classification.

[b]Sickness absence estimated from more highly aggregated disease classifications assuming days of absence are proportional to GP consultations within that class.

[c]Including £3·6 million for non-prescribed laxatives.

Source: Various official publications (see text) and Intercontinental Medical Statistics.

Individual Variation in Dietary Intake

Jean W. Marr

Royal Free Hospital, London

There are wide variations in energy and nutrient intakes *between* individuals. These have been shown for children (Widdowson, 1947; DHSS, 1975), for adults (Widdowson, 1936; Widdowson and McCance, 1936; Thomson, 1958) and for different occupational groups (Harries *et al.,* 1962). These examples all used the week's weighed inventory method of survey (Marr, 1971). The fact that variations exist between individuals enables groups to be identified within the distribution.

However, it is essential to establish that such variations do reflect the characteristics of the groups of individuals so identified and that the measurements are sufficiently valid for the purpose for which they are required (Rose and Blackburn, 1968). For instance, in the context of prevention related to nutrition it is important to be able to identify individuals or groups who may be at risk nutritionally either through inadequate intakes of particular nutrients or through excess. As well as the need for the measurements to be valid, the number of days to be included in any survey should also be considered for both aspects are important in achieving a "true" estimate of intakes.

Weekly variation within persons

To what extent intakes are stable for individuals from one week to another has been assessed by repeating the measurement. Different groups have shown varying degrees of stability over short periods, children and students being more variable (Huenemann and Turner, 1942; Yudkin, 1951) than adults (Thomson, 1958; Adelson, 1960; Morris *et al.,* 1963). However, for groups of individuals where seasonal patterns of physical activity are an important variable the variation in dietary intake may also show a seasonal variation (Keys *et al.,* 1966).

In adult men who showed considerable stability in intake from week to

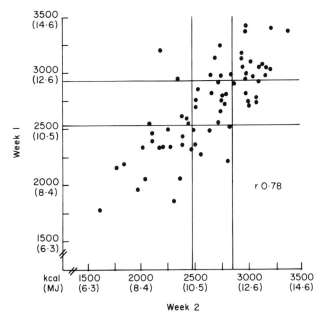

Figure 1   Energy intake for 68 men in two separate weeks.

week (Marr, 1971) it was possible to identify relatively stable individuals who were in the high or low thirds of the distribution on each of two separate weeks and the few individuals who were grossly different, i.e. in the top third of the distribution in one week, and the bottom in the other week, or vice versa (Fig. 1).

Daily variation, within persons

Intakes of individuals also vary from day to day. The degree of variation can be shown to affect the number of days for which it is necessary to record intakes in order to identify individuals as being in the extreme thirds of the distribution (Gardner and Heady, 1973) or the extreme fifths (Liu *et al.,* 1978).

Between- and within-person variation

The greater the between-person variation compared to the within-person variation, the shorter the period of recording that is necessary and vice versa. To illustrate this, data from two groups of male civil servants, aged

40−49 years, who weighed their food intake for 7 days in the autumn of 1970 and one group which repeated the survey in the spring of 1971 will be used. We can compare the within- and between-person variation and thus calculate the number of days it will be necessary to record (weigh) food intake in order to identify with a given precision the men in the high and low thirds of the distribution. Our aim would be to be 95% sure (Table I) that at least 80% are correctly classified and less than 1% grossly misclassified. The correlation coefficient between the "true" and "observed" values required for this is 0·90.

Table I

The number of days for which it is necessary to record (weigh) food intake in order to identify the men in the extreme thirds of the distribution so that 80% are correctly classified and less than 1% grossly misclassified $r = 0·90$. Based on data for three groups of male civil servants aged 40−49 years.

Group	A 83 men Oct./Nov. 1970	B 68 men Oct./Nov. 1970	B 68 men March 1971
Energy intake	7	7	6
Total protein	6	9	9
Total fat	9	8	10
Total carbohydrate	4	3	3
Total sugar	2	2	2
Dietary fibre	6	9	8
Dietary fibre from cereal sources	4	5	6
P/S ratio[a]	11	13	21
Dietary cholesterol	18	24	17
Alcohol	4	2	2

[a]Poly-unsaturated fatty acid to saturated fatty acid ratio.

How many days is it necessary to record (weigh) food intake?

For each nutrient the number of days for which it is necessary to record food intake show a remarkable degree of consistency for the three groups of men described in the previous section. The order of magnitude varies from around 20 days for dietary cholesterol, to about 2−3 days for total carbohydrate, sugar and alcohol. The reasons for these variations are the sources of the nutrient and the regularity with which the foods are eaten by the different subjects.

Dietary cholesterol, for instance, is present in small quantities in many foods but in very large quantities in a few foods which may not be eaten on a regular basis: there are thus large within-person or daily variations. The *P/S* ratio (poly-unsaturated to saturated fatty acid ratio) behaves in a similar manner and both these require many days recording in order to establish the level of consumption.

Total sugar (sugar taken in beverages as well as that used in cooked and made up dishes) on the other hand, shows much less within-person variation compared to the between-person variation and, therefore, relatively few days are needed to identify the men in the extreme thirds of the distribution.

Table II

The number of days for which it is necessary to record (weigh) food intake in order to identify the men in the extreme thirds of the distbribution — at varying degrees of correlation.

Group A: 83 men aged 40–49 years					
% correctly classified	69	72	76	80	86
% grossly misclassified	5	3	2	< 1	< 1
Correlation (*r*)	0·75	0·80	0·85	0·90	0·95
Energy intake	2	3	5	7	16
Total protein	2	3	4	6	14
Total fat	3	4	6	9	19
Total carbohydrate	2	2	3	4	9
Total sugar	1	1	2	2	5
Dietary fibre	2	3	4	6	12
Dietary fibre from cereal sources	2	2	3	4	8
P/S ratio	4	5	7	11	24
Dietary cholesterol	6	8	11	18	38
Alcohol	1	2	3	4	8

Table II demonstrates how the correlation coefficient behaves in relation to the percentage correctly classified and the number of days for which it is necessary to record intakes. Thus, in trying to identify the men in the extreme thirds of energy intake, if one uses a 3-day weighed record, about 70% will be correctly classified, whereas a 7-day record is needed to correctly classify 80% for this group of men, *r* being 0·90.

One day's intake

With data for one day derived from a weighed record it would be possible to correctly classify about 60% of individuals in the extreme thirds of the distribution for energy intake, protein, fat and dietary fibre, and about 10% would be grossly misclassified. The two groups of men are remarkably similar in this respect (Table III) for dietary cholesterol and the *P/S* ratio gross misclassification could be of the order of 15–20% and only about 50% would be correctly classified.

Table III

The percentage correctly classified and grossly misclassified when only a one-day weighed record is available. Two groups of civil servants: A (83 men), B (68 men).

	Groups	% correctly classified	% grossly misclassified
Energy intake	A	61	10
	B	62	9
Total protein	A	62	9
	B	59	11
Total fat	A	59	11
	B	60	10
Total carbohydrate	A	67	6
	B	70	4
Total sugar	A	74	2
	B	75	2
Dietary fibre	A	63	8
	B	59	11
Dietary fibre from cereal sources	A	67	6
	B	66	7
P/S ratio	A	55	14
	B	55	14
Dietary cholesterol	A	52	16
	B	50	18
Alcohol	A	68	5
	B	74	2

Discussion

For how many days is it necessary to keep a record? This will depend on the objectives of the study and the particular nutrients to be estimated. That the between- and within-person variations differ in respect of the different nutrients must be considered when deciding on the time period to be covered. Many investigators have tried to develop short-cut methods of dietary assessment for epidemiological surveys (Becker *et al.,* 1960; Wiehl and Reed, 1960; Marr *et al.,* 1961; Stefanik and Trulson, 1962; Hankin *et al.,* 1967). It would be highly desirable that such a method be based on a short time period with limited involvement of the subjects. Writing in 1959, Trulson and McCann concluded that "there is no technique for evaluating food intake that is practical for field conditions which gives a completely reliable pattern of the characteristic intake of the individual". In 1963, Abrahamson and others could not find a method that differentiated in terms of nutrients. In 1977, Morris *et al.* reported that they had "failed to find a valid and simple enough method suitable for large-scale study" and in 1978, Hankin *et al.* concluded that the short dietary method which they had developed, using frequency of use and average servings of food groups, showed a substantial lack of agreement between the observed and predicted intakes due to the variability among individuals in their eating habits.

Conclusion

Individuals vary in their dietary intakes one to another as well as within themselves from day to day. To identify those subjects at either end of the distribution for energy intake or for any given nutrient these variations must be taken into account.

References

Abramson, J. H., Slome, C. and Kosovsky, C. (1963) Food frequency interview as an epidemiological tool. *American Journal of Public Health,* **53,** 1093–101.

Adelson, S. F. (1960) Some problems in collecting dietary data from individuals. *Journal of the American Dietetic Association,* **36,** 453–61.

Becker, B. G., Indik, B. P. and Beeuwkes, A. M. (1960) "Dietary Intake Methodologies. A Review". Technical Report, University of Michigan.

DHSS (1975) "A Nutrition Survey of Pre-School Children, 1967–68", Report on Health and Social Subjects, 10. HMSO, London.

Gardner, M. J. and Heady, J. A. (1973) Some effects of within-person variability in epidemiological studies. *Journal of Chronic Diseases,* **26**, 781–95.

Hankin, J. H., Reynolds, W. E. and Margen, S. (1967) A short dietary method for epidemiological studies. *American Journal of Clinical Nutrition,* **20**, 935–45.

Hankin, J. H., Rawlings, V. and Nomura, A. (1978) Assessment of a short dietary method for a prospective study on cancer. *American Journal of Clinical Nutrition,* **31**, 355–9.

Harries, J. M., Hobson, E. A. and Hollingsworth, D. F. (1962) Individual variations in energy expenditure and intake. *Proceedings of the Nutrition Society,* **21**, 157–69.

Huenemann, R. L. and Turner, D. (1942) Methods of dietary investigation. *Journal of the American Dietetic Association,* **18**, 562–8.

Keys, A., Aravanis, C. and Sdrin, H. (1966) The diets of middle-aged men in two rural areas of Greece. *Voeding,* **27**, 575–86.

Liu, K., Stamler, J., Dyer, A., McKeever, J. and McKeever, P. (1978) Statistical methods to assess and minimize the role of intra-individual variability in obscuring the relationship between dietary lipids and serum cholesterol. *Journal of Chronic Diseases,* **31**, 399–418.

Marr, J. W., Heady, J. A. and Morris, J. N. (1961) Towards a method for large-scale individual diet surveys in, "Proceedings 3rd International Congress of Dietetics", pp. 85–90. Newman Books, London.

Marr, J. W. (1971) Individual dietary surveys: purposes and methods. *World Review of Nutrition and Dietetics,* **13**, 105–64.

Morris, J. N., Marr, J. W., Heady, J. A., Mills, G. L. and Pilkington, T. R. E. (1963) Diet and plasma cholesterol in 99 bankmen. *British Medical Journal,* **1**, 571–6.

Morris, J. N., Marr, J. W. and Clayton, D. G. (1977) Diet and heart: a postscript. *British Medical Journal,* **2**, 1307–14.

Rose, G. A. and Blackburn, H. (1968) "Cardiovascular Survey Methods". World Health Organization, Geneva.

Stefanik, P. A. and Trulson, M. F. (1962) Determining the frequency intakes of foods in large group studies. *American Journal of Clinical Nutrition,* **11**, 335–43.

Thomson, A. M. (1958) Diet in pregnancy. *British Journal of Nutrition,* **12**, 446–61.

Trulson, M. F. and McCann, M. B. (1959) Comparison of dietary survey methods. *Journal of the American Dietetic Association,* **35**, 672–6.

Widdowson, E. M. (1936) A study of English diets by the individual method, part 1, men. *Journal of Hygiene,* **36**, 269–92.

Widdowson, E. M. and McCance, R. A. (1936) A study of English diets by the individual method, II, women. *Journal of Hygiene,* **36**, 293–309.

Widdowson, E. M. (1947) "A Study of Individual Children's Diets", Special Report No. 257, Medical Research Council. HMSO, London.

Wiehl, D. G. and Reed, R. (1960) Development of new or improved dietary methods for epidemiological investigations. *American Journal of Public Health,* **50**, 824–8.

Yudkin, J. (1951) Dietary surveys: variation in the weekly intake of nutrients. *British Journal of Nutrition,* **4**, 177–94.

The Role of Diet in the Prevention of Dental Caries

Malcolm N. Naylor

Department of Periodontology and Preventive Dentistry,
Guy's Hospital Dental School, London

The role of diet in preventing dental caries

Dental caries is a disease of microbial origin, insidious in onset and slow in its progress. Once the disease has passed beyond its very early stages it is irreversible and can only be treated by surgical means. This involves removal of the diseased tissue and its replacement by a metal or plastic filling material or the extraction of the tooth.

Dental caries is essentially a disease of the human race though under special circumstances it can be induced in certain species, notably rat and monkey. Such animals require highly specialized diets vastly differing from their natural foods; in some instances it is necessary to inoculate the mouth of the animal with specific caries-associated micro-organisms. Most animals, including dog and cat, appear totally incapable of developing carious lesions.

In western civilization the prevalence of dental caries is high. Indeed, it has been estimated that by age 15 years, 97% of young people in the UK have an average 10 out of their 23 teeth either decayed, filled or extracted. (Todd, 1975). There is, however, growing evidence that the situation is improving. For example, in 1963, 37% of a carefully compiled random sample of the population aged 16 years and over wore full upper and lower dentures. More recently Beal and Dowell (1977) have shown that this percentage has fallen to 31%. The recently published report by Todd and Walker (1980) on the state of adult dental health between 1968 and 1978 confirm this improvement.

Because of its irreversible nature and its widespread prevalence, for many years there have been attempts to devise methods to prevent and control dental caries. Early procedures were empirically based but as a clearer understanding of the cause and natural history of the disease emerged, decay prevention methods have become increasingly rational.

It was towards the end of the last century that W. D. Miller first enunciated the chemico-parasitic theory of dental caries (Miller, 1890). Although this theory was derived from a series of very simple and crude test-tube experiments, it nevertheless provided a firm basis for a wealth of subsequent work which has been carried out and is continuing in many countries throughout the world.

As has been stated already, dental caries is primarily a microbial disease. However, there are many secondary factors involved and amongst these, dietary influences are perhaps the most important.

Micro-organisms of many kinds colonize on tooth surfaces which are not readily cleansed by the action of the mobile soft tissue structures of the mouth. These colonies coalesce to form plaques which comprise dense accumulations of bacteria bound together and firmly adherent to the tooth surface by means of extra-cellular polysaccharides, mainly of the glucan type. The microbial composition of plaque varies from individual to individual but, generally speaking, young plaque is made up of Gram-positive, aerobic coccal forms, whereas older plaque comprises mainly Gram-negative, anaerobic rod-shaped forms.

The micro-organisms undergo metabolic activity, the nature of which depends upon the substrate provided by the dietary intake. Many plaque organisms are capable of breaking down sugars to form organic acids capable of "attacking" enamel surfaces. Of the various mono- and disaccharides in the diet, sucrose is of especial importance.

Plaque micro-organism enzyme systems appear to be capable of metabolizing sucrose in two ways. First, sucrose is broken down anaerobically to form lactic acid which accumulates and lowers the pH at the plaque–enamel interface sufficiently for the tooth surface to be attacked. Second, sucrose units can be polymerized to form extracellular polysaccharides, mainly of the glucan type. These polysaccharides serve to provide substrate material to the micro-organisms between food intake. In addition, they cause the plaque to thicken and so reduce plaque-permeability to salivary buffer systems. Thus the state of diffusion of salivary buffers is insufficient to neutralize acids accumulating at the plaque–tooth interface.

Caries begins as a sub-surface demineralization of the enamel and it is only when the lesion has extended considerably that collapse of the surface occurs and actual cavitation becomes identifiable. It has been estimated that a period of between 18 and 24 months may elapse between initiation of the lesion and its clinical recognition (Parfitt, 1956). In older individuals the process may be even slower. Indeed, Emslie (1963) reported that radiologically demonstrated interproximal lesions showed no evidence of progressive enlargement over a two-year period.

Caries prevention

A modern practical approach to caries prevention is multifactorial and includes effective removal of microbial plaque, dietary control and the appropriate use of fluorides.

Although the nature of dental caries makes it extremely difficult, both from the ethical and scientific point of view, to design and carry out controlled human studies there is a wealth of evidence relating the disease with the consumption of carbohydrate-containing foods.

It was Miller (1890) who firmly established this relationship when he obtained caries-like lesions in extracted teeth which had been incubated in human saliva in the presence of carbohydrate.

There are numerous instances of primitive communities abandoning their well established natural diet in favour of the softened and refined diets of civilized man, with a concomitant increase in caries experience. Examples include the Bantu tribes of South Africa (Oranje *et al.*, 1935), Eskimos (Curzon and Curzon, 1970), Greenlanders (Pedersen, 1938), and the islanders of Tristan da Cuhna (Holloway *et al.*, 1963).

Of course when such drastic changes in diet occur, a number of factors may be involved. These include the loss of possible protective substances in the diet and an effect on the development and maturation of the teeth themselves. For example, when the Eskimo changed his diet not only did his sugar intake increase but his intake of fat decreased considerably (Pigman, 1970).

The whole question of "protective factors" and possible influence of dietary changes on tooth development and maturation are matters which require further investigation.

During the Second World War the amount of sugar consumed in many European countries was considerably reduced and there were a number of reports of consequent reductions in the prevalence of dental caries (Toverud, 1949). However, in one investigation (King *et al.*, 1955), twice and three times the normal amount of sugar was included in the diet of institutionalized children of various ages. After one and two years there were no differences in the incidence of caries between control and experimental groups.

Perhaps the most important study to date has been that carried out at the Vipeholm Hospital, Sweden (Gustafson *et al.*, 1954). In this study 436 inmates of the hospital, a long-stay institution, were placed on closely controlled and specified diets and observed for a period of 5 years. The study comprised seven groups, the first three of which ate carbohydrates at meal times only; the remaining four groups supplemented their diet by between-meal consumption of sweets.

The groups were designated as follows:

1. Control group   This group received a fully nutritional basic diet with an energy supplement in the form of margarine.

2. Sucrose group   This group was provided daily with 300 g of sucrose in solution for 2 years, after which the amount was reduced to 75 g.

3. Bread group   This group was given 345 g of sweetened bread which provided 50 g of sucrose a day. The addition of the sugar made the bread somewhat sticky when chewed.

4. Chocolate group   For the first 2 years of the study, this group received sucrose in solution, but for the remaining 2 years they received 65 g of milk chocolate daily to be eaten between meals.

5. Caramel group   This group received 22 caramels per day which contained a total of 70 g of sucrose. These were given in four batches of 4 or 5 sweets at a time throughout the day.

6. 8-Toffee group   This group was provided with 8 toffees per day containing a total of 60 g of sucrose. They were eaten between meals for a 3-year period.

7. 24-Toffee group   This group was given 24 toffees daily to be eaten between meals. These provided 120 g of sucrose per day. The study extended over 18 months.

The overall findings of this study indicate that the consumption of sucrose can increase caries experience but that the risk is greatly enhanced if the sucrose is given in a sticky form which is consumed between meals. It also demonstrated that the withdrawal of such foodstuffs from the diet caused the high caries susceptibility to subside.

Another interesting finding was that caries activity differed widely from subject to subject even under strictly controlled dietary regimens. Furthermore, despite avoidance of sticky sucrose-containing foods and other natural sugars, some subjects continued to have new carious lesions, albeit at a low rate.

Although the design and conduct of this study are open to criticism it must be remembered that it is the only long-term longitudinal study carried out under precisely controlled conditions. Amongst the criticisms are the small size of the study groups, the high average age of the groups, the poor plaque control and the general low mentality of the subjects. Despite those defects, all of which would militate against differences being shown, the study clearly demonstrates that it is not so much the quantity of sucrose consumed which is important but rather the frequency of eating and stickiness of form.

Other studies, less well controlled and covering shorter periods of time, have supported the Vipeholm findings:

a) Zita *et al.* (1959) studied the food intake over one week of 200 children aged 5–13 years and showed a positive correlation between the amount of sugar-containing foods eaten between meals and caries prevalence. There was no correlation between total sugar consumption and caries prevalence.

b) Similar findings were reported by Weiss and Trithart (1960) in a study of a one-day dietary intake of 783 children aged 4–5 years.

c) Mansbridge (1960), however, found that in 12- to 14-year-old children it was necessary to consume 230 g or more of sweets or chocolate per week in order to obtain more decay than those who ate none.

d) In a longitudinal study Harris (1963) found that the caries level in a group of children in an institution on a vegetarian and dairy product diet without added refined carbohydrate was only about 10% of that in the general population. When the children left the institution caries soon developed.

e) Fanning *et al.* (1969) showed that in schools with facilities available for the purchase of sweets, the children had a higher caries experience than in those schools where such facilities did not exist.

f) Extensive and rapid carious breakdown of the deciduous anterior teeth of babies and young children is a feature commonly associated with the use of sweetened drinks fed by means of reservoir-type feeders. Such drinks, which may be sweetened milk or undiluted syrups, are often given at night time as a "comforter" to induce and maintain sleep. Certainly on the grounds of prevention of caries this is a dietary practice much to be deprecated.

Sucrose substitutes

In recent years there have been attempts to introduce into the diet sweetening agents other than sucrose. These have fallen into the two basic categories: (a) low calorie sweeteners and (b) calorific sweeteners.

Of the non-calorific agents, saccharin is the one most widely used in the home, by the food industry and by dentifrice manufacturers. Cyclamates were of course an alternative until their general withdrawal a decade or so ago.

Calorific sweeteners have been studied extensively and animal studies (Guggenheim *et al.*, 1966) have indicated that replacement of sucrose by mono- and disaccharides such as glucose, maltose and lactose causes considerable reduction in caries experience. Human studies, which are extremely difficult to control with the same precision as animal studies, have failed to confirm these reductions in man.

However, sweets and toffees made with sorbitol, mannitol or Lycasin as the sweetening agent do not reduce plaque pH to below 5·7 (Imfeld and Mühlemann, 1977) and thus have been designated in Switzerland as *Kariesschonend* (tooth protective).

Perhaps the most exciting sucrose substitute which has been investigated recently is xylitol, a polyhydric sugar alcohol derived from wood pulp. In a series of investigations, now known collectively as the Turku Sugar Studies, it has been convincingly demonstrated that xylitol in human diets is less cariogenic than either sucrose or fructose (Scheinin *et al.*, 1976). Xylitol occurs naturally in a number of foods, including bananas and mushrooms and has a degree of sweetness similar to sucrose. A limiting factor to its use would appear to be that, as with sorbitol, it can cause an osmotic diarrhoea, and at the present time is costly.

Trace elements

For many years attempts have been made to relate the intake of trace elements with dental caries experience. Considerable difficulty has been encountered in such studies because of the biological interaction between one particular ion and others in the diet. For example, it was shown by Adler (1953) that in areas where the molybdenum intake was higher, the caries incidence was reduced. This and other studies failed to take into account the effect on molybdenum of such dietary trace elements as copper, manganese and vanadium; this may well account for the contradictary findings between studies.

Other elements which may affect caries prevalence include selenium, which appears to cause it to rise, and iron, strontium and lithium which seem to cause it to fall. The highly complex interrelationships between caries prevalence and dietary trace-element intake has been discussed by Curzon (1977).

Fluoride

Undoubtedly the most effective practical measure available at the present time for reducing the caries prevalence in the community is the provision of an optimum amount of dietary fluoride. Fluorine is an ubiquitous element and is present in varying trace amounts in virtually all drinking-water supplies. Dean *et al.* (1942) in a study of almost 8000 children domiciled in twenty-one US cities with fluoride levels in their water supplies varying from near zero to 2·6 ppm, showed an inverse relationship between caries prevalence and the fluoride level. This relationship has been amply confirmed by many subsequent studies carried out in other parts of the world and as a consequence schemes were devised to adjust the level in drinking-water to 1 ppm of the fluoride ion (F⁻), the indicated optimal level. The first such scheme began in 1945 at Grand Rapids (Knuston, 1970) and after 10 years the caries prevalence had fallen by over 50% (Arnold *et al.,* 1956). Subsequent studies in the USA (Ast *et al.,* 1956; Blayney and Hill, 1967), in Canada (Hutton *et al.,* 1951; Brown and Poplove, 1965), in Holland (Kwant *et al.,* 1969) and in the UK (DHSS, 1969) all confirmed the Grand Rapid findings.

The process of adjusting the fluoride ion level in drinking-water supplies is known as fluoridation. The addition of fluoride ions carried out at the water works by means of a fluoridator which operates on a fail-safe basis. Further, by incorporating into the system a specific ion electrode, continuous monitoring of the fluoride ion (F⁻) level is achieved.

At the present time 108 million citizens of the USA drink water with a fluoride ion content of approximately 1 ppm. Of these, 97 million consume water in which the fluoride ion level has been adjusted by fluoridation. The remainder live in areas with "natural" fluoride in the water (Whitford, 1980). In the UK, the situation is less satisfactory. Whilst fluoridation has been endorsed for many years by successive governments, the Royal Colleges, professional associations and many other bodies, its progress has been disappointingly slow. Indeed of the major cities only in Birmingham and Newcastle upon Tyne is the public water supply at present fluoridated.

Conclusions

Dental caries is primarily a microbial disease but dietary factors play an essential role in the initiation and progress of a lesion. Furthermore, the disease can be controlled and prevented by dietary means. These comprise modification of the patterns of consumption of dietary carbohydrates, notably sucrose and the inclusion in the diet, especially during the tooth-forming years, of an adequate amount of fluoride ion. Dietary fluoride can be provided in a number of ways, but adjustment of the level in the public drinking-water supplies would seem to be the safest and most effective way of ensuring that the benefit reaches the community as a whole.

In the final analysis the prevention of dental caries requires far-reaching changes in personal habits, not least dietary habits. To bring about these changes every preventive programme must contain a major educational component in which the value of a healthy intact dentition is stressed. Until the community appreciate to the full the benefits of good oral health in terms of function and aesthetics, and accept that a "natural dentition for life" is well within the reach of everyone, progress will be limited.

Perhaps therefore, the most important step forward will be to establish educational programmes amongst the most sensitive and vulnerable parts of the community—children, pregnant women and nursing mothers. The dental profession alone cannot shoulder this task. It requires a much broader approach and must include the health professions, including nutritionists, government, industry and the public. Indeed, it is a community responsibility.

References

Adler, P. (1953) A water-borne caries-protective agent other than fluoride. *Med. Acad. Sci. Hung.,* **4**, 221–6.

Arnold, F. A., Dean, H. T., Jay, P. and Knuston, J. W. (1956) Effect of fluoridated public water supplies on dental caries prevalence. 10th year of the Grand Rapids–Muskegons study. *Pub. Hlth Rep.,* **71**, 652–8.

Ast, D. B., Smith, D. J., Wacks, B. and Cantwell, K. W. (1956) Newburgh–Kingston caries fluoride study XIV. Combined clinical and roentgenographic findings after 10 years of fluoride experience. *J. Am. Dent. Ass.,* **52**, 314–25.

Beal, J. F. and Dowell, T. B. (1977) Edentulousness and attendance patterns in England and Wales. *Brit. dent. J.* **143**, 203–307.

Blayney, J. R. and Hill, I. N. (1967) Fluoride and dental caries. *J. Am. Dent. Ass.,* **74**, 233–302.

Brown, H. K. and Poplove, M. (1965) Brantford–Sarnia–Stratford fluoridation caries studies: final survey. 1963 *J. Canad. Dent. Ass.,* **31**, 505–11.

Curzon, M. and Curzon, J. A. (1970) Dental caries in Eskimo children of the Keetwatin District of the Northwestern Territories. *J. Canad. Dent. Ass.,* **36**, 342–5.

Curzon, M. J. (1977) "Trace element composition of human enamel on dental caries". Ph.D. Thesis, University of London.

Dean, H. T., Arnold, F. A. and Elvove, E. (1942) Domestic water and dental caries *Pub. Hlth Rep.,* **57**, 1155–79.

Department of Health and Social Security (1969) Report of the committee on research into fluoridation. The fluoridation studies in the United Kingdom and the results achieved after eleven years. *Rep. Pub. Hlth Med. Subj.* No. 122. HMSO, London.

Emslie, R. D. (1963) Clinical trial of a toothpaste containing sarcosinates (Abstr.). *J. dent. Res.,* **42**, 1079.

Fanning, E. A., Gotjamandos, T. and Vowles, N. J. (1969) Dental caries in children related to availability of sweets at school canteens. *Med. J. Austr.,* **1**, 1131–2.

Guggenheim, B. B., Konig, K. G., Hertzog, G. and Muhlemann, H. R. (1966) The cariogenicity of different dietary carbohydrates tested on rats in relative guotobiosis with a streptococcus producing extra-cellular polysaccharides. *Helv. Acta,* **10**, 101–13.

Gustafsson, B. E., Quensel, C. E., Lanke, L. S., Lundquist, C. Grahnen, H., Bonow, B. E. and Krasse, B. (1954) The Vipeholm dental caries study: the effect of different levels of carbohydrate intake on caries activity in 436 individuals observed for 5 years. *Acta odont. Scand.,* **11**, 232–363.

Harris, R. (1963) Biology of the children of Hopewood House, Bowral, Australia. 4. Observations of dental caries experience extending over 5 years (1957–1961). *J. dent. Res.,* **42**, 1387–98.

Holloway, P. J., James, P. M. C. and Slack, G. L. (1963) Dental disease in Tristan da Cunha. *Brit. dent. J.,* **115**, 19–25.

Hutton, W. L., Linscott, B. W. and Williams, D. B. (1951) Brantford fluoride experiment *Can. J. Pub. Hlth.,* **42**, 81–9.

Imfeld, T. and Mühlemann, H. R. (1977) Evaluation of sugar substitute in preventative cariology. *J. prev. Dent.,* **4**, 8–14.

King, J. D., Mellanby, M., Stones, H. H. and Green, H. N. (1955) "The Effect of Sugar Supplements on Dental Caries in Children". Medical Research Council Special Report Series No. 288. HMSO, London.

Knuston, J. W. (1970) Water fluoridation after 25 years. *Brit. dent. J.,* **129**, 297–300.

Kwant, G. W., Howink, B. and Backer-Dirks, O. (1969) Fluoridetoevoeging aan drinkwater. 3. Resulten van het onderzoek Tiel-colomborg na 13 and one half jaar. *Nederl. T. Tandheelk,* **76**, 281–302.

Mansbridge, J. T. (1960) The effects of oral hygiene and sweet consumption on the prevalence of dental caries. *Brit. dent. J.,* **109**, 343–8.

Miller, W. D. (1890) "The Micro-organisms of the Human Mouth". S. S. White, Philadelphia.

Oranje, P., Noriskin, J. N., and Osborn, T. B. W. (1935) The effects of diet upon dental caries in South African Bantu. *Sth Afr. J. Med. Sci.,* **1**, 57–62.

Parfitt, G. J. (1956) The speed and development of the carious cavity. *Brit. dent. J.* **100**, 204–7.

Pedersen, P. O. (1938) Investigation of dental conditions of about 3,000 ancient and modern Greenlanders—a preliminary report. *Dent. Rec.,* **58**, 191–8.

Pigman, W. (1970) Carbohydrates, fats and dental caries. *Adv. Chem. Serv.,* **94**, 7–22.

Scheinin, A., Makinen, K. K. and Ylitalo, K. (1976) Turku Sugar Studies V. Final report on the effect of sucrose, fructose and xylitol diets on the caries incidence in man. *Acta. odont. Scand.,* **34**, 179–216.

Todd, J. E. (1975) "Children's Dental Health in England and Wales 1973". Office of Population Census and Surveys, HMSO, London.

Todd, J. E. (1980) "Adult Dental Health, Vol. 1: England and Wales 1968–1978". Office of Population Census and Surveys, HMSO, London.

Toverud, G. (1949) Dental caries in Norwegian children during and after the last world war. *Proc. roy. Soc. Med., **42**, 249–58.*

Weiss, R. L. and Trithart, A. H. (1960) Between meal eating habits and dental caries experience in pre-school children. *Am. J. Publ. Hlth, **50**, 1097–104.*

Whitford, G. M. (1980) People and events. *J. Am. Dent. Ass., **100**, 413–4.*

Zita, C., McDonald, R. E. and Andrews, A. L. (1959) Dietary habits and dental caries experience in 200 children. *J. dent. Res., **38**, 860–5.*

The Influence of Social Environment on the Nutrition of Mother and Child

Eva Alberman

The London Hospital Medical College, London

It is not easy to know how best to assess the nutritional status of a population. Measurements of food intake, either qualitative or quantitative, are notoriously difficult to carry out in large samples of individuals over any length of time. Moreover such measures do not necessarily reflect the amount of food which is actually absorbed or utilized; but utilization studies are even more difficult to carry out, particularly on large numbers of individuals. Calorie needs too vary with many factors, including body build and physical activity. All these considerations make a direct assessment of the nutritional status of a population exceedingly difficult, a problem which has been discussed by Rush in 1975. In practice the most common indicators of nutritional status used in population studies are birthweight, ultimate height and rate of growth, weight, and other anthropometric measures. There is now abundant evidence to show that these are associated with past or present dietary intake and socio-economic status. These associations have been very extensively researched and I cannot hope to do more than to present an outline of such published work in the field of maternal and child health. Much of this work has been reviewed in a recently published series on human growth edited by Faulkner and Tanner (1978).

Social factors and birthweight

The distribution of birthweight in a population is considerably affected by social as well as biological cirumstances. Studies all over the world have shown how, within a given population, birthweight falls with social disadvantage; examples are given in Table I from the two most recent British national studies (Butler and Alberman, 1969; Chamberlain *et al.*, 1975).

Table I

Mean birthweight (g) by social
class (National Birthday Trust
Studies, 1958, 1970).

| Social class | Year of birth | |
	1958	1970
I	3400 ⎫	
II	3375 ⎬	3377
III	3320	3356
IV	3320 ⎫	
V	3290 ⎬	3264

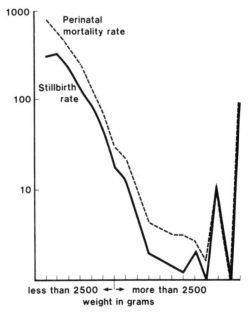

Figure 1   Perinatal mortality rate and stillbirth rate per 1000 total births (log scale) by birthweight group, Greater Manchester, 1978. (Evidence to Parliamentary Social Services Committee from North West Regional Hospital Board, 1980.)

The significance of birthweight

The significance of birthweight is far-reaching. It is strongly associated with risk of perinatal mortality and of some handicapping disorders, and with later growth.

Perinatal mortality falls sharply with birthweight up to about 4500 g (Fig. 1). Indeed the level of perinatal mortality in a geographical area, or in a country, is largely determined by distribution of birthweight. A recent WHO study (1978) showed that the rank order of countries by perinatal mortality rates changed substantially when birthweight distribution was taken into account, and the same has been shown to be true for Area Health Authorities in this country (Mallett and Knox, 1979).

Certain handicapping disorders also are more common in survivors of low birthweight, in particular spastic diplegia, and other forms of cerebral palsy (MacDonald, 1964), and almost certainly there is some positive relationship between fetal growth rate and intellectual performance, although it is practically impossible to disentangle this effect satisfactorily from post-natal influences.

Genetic factors and birthweight

There are certainly some genetic and other inherent factors determining ultimate birthweight and rate of fetal growth, although it is often very difficult to disentangle these from environmental effects, particularly when the importance of ethnic group in determining birthweight is considered. The latter question has been extensively studied in the USA where, as in so many countries, the minority ethnic groups are also most often suffering from socio-economic disadvantage. It is well-known that in the USA black babies are of lower birthweight than white babies of the same gestational age and this seems to be true in every occupational group (Garn *et al*, 1977). Black mothers also have a shorter gestational period than white. Garn and Bailey (1978) have produced elegant evidence from cross-racial marriages suggesting that the latter effect is determined more by the mother than the father (Table II).

Table II

Gestational "prematurity" (≤37 weeks) in intraracial and interracial marriages; live born singletons (Garn *et al.*, 1977).

Parental combination			
Mother	Father	No.	Per cent 37 weeks gestation
Black	Black	9901	26·2
Black	White	34	20·6
White	Black	98	17·3
White	White	9433	11·7

Maternal stature and diet and birthweight

Table III shows the relationship between maternal height and birthweight in the National Birthday Trust national birth surveys (Butler and Alberman, 1969; Chamberlain *et al.*, 1975) demonstrating how birthweight rises with increasing maternal height. From the 1958 survey data it was possible to show that, even within social class, birthweight increases with maternal height. In an earlier study Professor Thomson (1959) had looked at maternal height, weight, calorie intake and birthweight. He concluded that although these were all associated with each other maternal weight was more important in the prediction of birthweight than either height or calorie intake, and that the influence of current diet on birthweight must be very small. These conclusions have been confirmed by many other workers (Metcoff, 1978).

Table III

Mean birth weight by maternal height group; singletons of 38—41 weeks' gestation (National Birthday Trust Studies, 1958, 1970).

Maternal height group (inches)	Mean birth weight (g) 1958 study	1970 study
61 and under	3241	3232
62—64	3350	3362
65 and over	3486	3473

The only studies which have shown that current diet is of importance in the prediction of birthweight are those carried out on mothers suffering from acute or chronic malnutrition. Stein, Susser and their colleagues (1975) investigated the outcome of pregnancies occurring during the wartime famine in Holland. They were able to show that mean birthweight was reduced in mothers pregnant during the famine, but the effect was found only in pregnancies exposed in the third trimester of pregnancy. This was in a population in whom previous nutrition had been good, and where nutrition rapidly returned to an adequate level after the famine. In a series of studies on mothers with chronic malnutrition in rural parts of Guatemala (Lechtig *et al.*, 1975) it is claimed that food supplementation during pregnancy actually increased birthweight, although it was not possible to carry out a randomized control trial. Susser and his colleagues (Susser and Stein, 1977) carried out a randomized control trial of nutritional intervention in a group of black pregnant mothers known to be at high risk of low birthweight. They found that only in women of a pre-pregnant weight of under 110 pounds and in those who smoked did a nutritional supplement increase birthweight, and indeed there was a small unexpected excess of premature deliveries in the supplemented group.

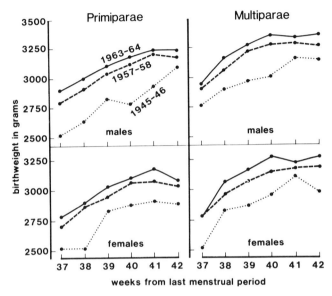

Figure 2 Mean birthweight by gestational age, Japan 1945−6, 1957−8 and 1963−4 (Gruenwald *et al.*, 1967).

However there are data from Japan (Fig. 2) (Gruenwald *et al.*, 1967) to show that birthweight distribution of a population can be increased in a relatively short time by an improvement in standards of living, as occurred in post-war Japan. We may conclude that although birthweight is certainly reduced in poor socio-economic circumstances, this is generally not accounted for by deficiencies in diet during pregnancy, except in conditions of extreme deprivation. In fact the data from the 1958 British Perinatal Mortality Survey (Butler and Alberman, 1969) showed that maternal height differences alone accounted for the association of low social class with reduced birthweight.

There is currently considerable interest in the possibility that specific deficiencies, or toxins, in maternal diet may be associated with an increased risk of bearing a child with a neural tube defect (Renwick, 1972; Smithells *et al.*, 1980). These suggestions are supported by the finding from Stein *et al.*

(1975) that this specific risk was increased in children exposed *in utero* to the Dutch famine and from Sir Dugald Baird's demonstration (1977) that it was more common in babies born to a cohort of mothers themselves born during a period of economic depression.

Birth order and birthweight

There are other associations with birthweight which are themselves linked with social circumstances. In our society the type of mother who goes on to have many pregnancies is, in general, at higher than average risk of low birthweight babies possibly because she is more likely to be of low social class; the mothers who have only few and widely spaced pregnancies are at lower than average risk (Bakketeig and Hoffman, 1979). Nevertheless both groups show some increase in birthweight with increasing birth order, particularly from the first to the second pregnancy, an effect which seems to be biologically determined.

Smoking and birthweight

The other socially determined association with birthweight which is of major importance is maternal smoking. By now the evidence is overwhelming that smoking is a cause of low birthweight. The more cigarettes smoked in pregnancy the lower the average birthweight, even with a homogenous social class, as in a group of women doctors (Table IV) (Alberman *et al.*, 1977). There is also some evidence that mothers who

Table IV

Mean birthweight (g) of singletons in relation to maternal smoking (Alberman *et al.*, 1977).

Parity	Cigarettes/day at time of conception		
	0	1−10	11+
0	3345	3254	3248
1	3437	3364	3332
2	3491	3418	3395
3+	3467	3521	3537
All	3410	3329	3324

smoke in very early pregnancy are at higher than average risk of spontaneous abortion, but this evidence is not as strong as that for its effect on birthweight (Kline *et al.*, 1977). The question of whether the effect of smoking on birthweight is mediated through a reduction of food intake in smokers, or whether it is purely secondary to a toxic effect of products of cigarette smoking, or to a combination of both, is still not fully answered. It is probably a combination of both.

Amongst other factors lowering birthweight are maternal hypertension, infections, and congenital disorders, but there are still many births of low weight which are quite unexplained.

Social factors and growth in infancy and later childhood

The very rapid growth seen in neonates and infants is largely determined by food intake and is outside the scope of the present paper. However later in childhood, growth is affected by many social factors including those mentioned earlier, and Fig. 3 shows the magnitude of some of these effects in a cross-sectional study (Davie *et al.*, 1972). It seems likely that some of

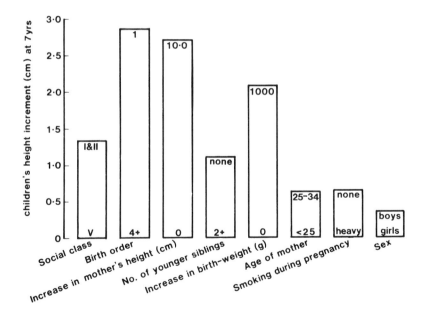

Figure 3   Increment in height at 7 years in children of different socio-biological background, National Child Development Study (Davie *et al.*, 1972).

these factors, like size of family and position in family, are mediated through their effect on the family budget and therefore food purchases, but the effects are certainly more complex than this alone.

Social factors seem to affect both ultimate stature and growth rate, and also affect the age at which puberty is reached. Thus Eveleth and Tanner (1976) have shown that the age of puberty tends to be earlier in urban areas than in rural, and there seems to have been a fall in mean age at puberty over the years all over the world, although in the most developed countries the rate of this fall has been decreasing (Fig. 4, Tanner, 1978). There also seem to be real ethnic differences in the ages at which puberty is reached.

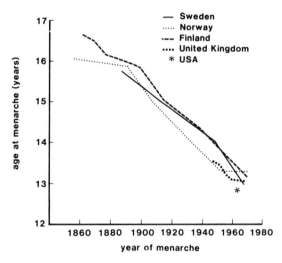

Figure 4   Mean age at menarche in selected countries 1860–1980 (from Tanner, 1978).

Many other factors have been shown to affect growth rate. Psychosocial factors can affect growth rate even in the presence of sufficient nutrient intake (Widdowson, 1951) as can congenital defects such as Down syndrome; the season of the year and certainly infections or other illness, particularly in association with poor nutrition.

Rate of growth at any age is of course affected directly by nutrition. Tanner (1978) gives examples of the heights of German schoolchildren falling during the First and Second World Wars, and rising between the wars. This, together with other abundant evidence outlined below, suggests that the association of poor socio-economic status with short stature is causal and is directly or indirectly related to nutrition.

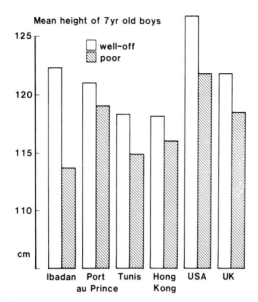

Figure 5 Mean height of 7 year-old boys, well-off and poor, in samples from different countries (from Eveleth: in Tanner and Falkner, 1978).

Firstly in every country but one in which this has been studied, disadvantaged children are smaller than those in the privileged classes, even though there are often substantial inter-country differences (Eveleth, 1978; Fig. 5). The one example where this does not seem to be true is present day urban Sweden, where a recent study has shown no difference in height of children by fathers' occupation (Lindgren, 1976). Tanner (1978) interprets this as an example of a classless society.

Seondly many international studies have shown that, with improving socio-economic circumstances over time, the height distributions of whole populations have shifted so that average height in children and adults has increased over the years (Fig. 6). This change seems to have been particularly rapid in Japan from 1950 to 1970, where an increase of height of 7-year-olds amounted to 3 cm/decade, and of 12-year-olds 5 cm/decade (Tanner, 1978).

Thirdly, studies of migrants from poorer to richer countries have shown that the immigrants tend to grow taller than those remaining at home. Kagan *et al.* (1974) shows how the height of adult Japanese males whose families migrated to California and Hawaii was greater than of the indigenous Japanese. However, later studies show that in Japan itself the rapid increase in stature has meant that the differences between growth of

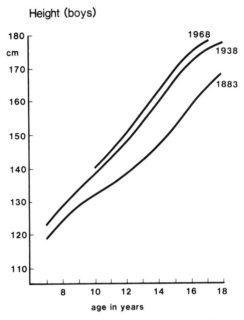

Height (boys)

Figure 6 Mean height at different ages of a sample of boys in Sweden, 1883, 1938 and 1968 (from Tanner, 1978).

children born more recently to migrants and to the indigenous group have virtually disappeared (Tanner, 1978).

Table V shows that in the 1960s the difference in adult height in migrants and indigenous Japanese was associated with differences of total calorie intake, and qualitative differences in diet, and indeed also with differences in serum cholesterol and blood pressure.

Table V

Mean dietary values (24-h recall) and biochemical characteristics. Japanese in California, Hawaii and Japan (Kagan *et al.*, 1974).

	Japan	Hawaii	California
Calories	2132	2274	2268
Total protein (g)	76	94	89
Total fat (g)	36	85	95
Total carbohydrate (g)	336	260	251
Cholesterol (mg/100 ml) at age 45−49 years	176·3	219·4	223·4
Systolic blood pressure (mmHg) at age 45−49 years	125·7	128·6	133·5

Ultimate adult height must be determined by the interaction between growth rate and age at skeletal maturity, and it seems that the latter also can be delayed in the presence of malnutrition. However, with long-standing malnutrition skeletal maturation occurs before full potential growth is achieved. The secular increase of adult height that was mentioned earlier in this paper has presumably come about by reversing this process through improvements in social conditions, so that maximum potential growth is achieved before skeletal maturation is completed.

Significance of growth rate and ultimate growth achieved

The significance of stunted growth has been much debated. Certainly it is not reasonable to extrapolate from one race to another, or one country to another. Tanner (1978) has pointed out that differences in body shapes and sizes may be needed to adapt to different climates or cultures. Nevertheless within a country and an ethnic group small stature is most often indicative of disadvantage and tends to be accompanied by higher risks of ill-health of most kinds, including a higher risk of perinatal mortality within each social class group (Fig. 7).

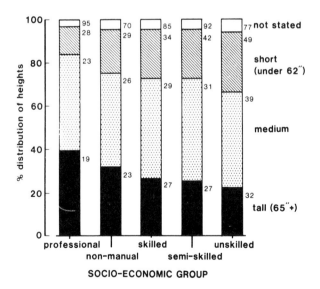

Figure 7 Distribution of maternal height by social class, and perinatal mortality rate in each group (National Birthday Trust Perinatal Mortality Study, 1958).

The most highly debated issue has been whether a stunting of post-natal growth is a cause of a reduction in mental ability. This question is particularly difficult to answer since the deprivations that lead to a nutritional deficit sufficient to slow down normal growth are almost inevitably accompanied by other forms of cultural or psychological deprivation. At the least these may be due to an affected child being too weak to explore its surroundings in the same way as a well-nourished child. Moreover there is general agreement that the effects of nutritional deprivation in the post-natal period will depend on the nutritional status of the child at birth, the length of time of post-natal deprivation, and probably on the stimulation it receives during and after the period of malnutrition. There is also considerable evidence to suggest that there are periods in development when the brain is relatively more or less vulnerable to malnutrition (Dobbing, 1976). These problems are discussed at length by various contributors to Falkner and Tanner (1978).

Obesity

Finally I should mention the problem of obesity, which is the major public health nutritional worry in the developed countries. Without question this is closely related to the level of education of a population, and should be one of the major targets of our health educators. I cannot here go into the evidence showing the health risks that obesity confers but I am sure you are all fully aware of these.

Conclusion

In summary the state of nutrition of a population has often been assessed by anthropometric measures. Nutritional status, measured in this way, is highly sensitive to socio-economic factors, although these are not always directly related to diet. Over the years improvements in socio-economic conditions in the developed countries have resulted in a general increase in stature, but even now socio-economic differences within a population are associated with differences in stature and health risk. More subtle influences on nutritional status are psychosocial state, and factors such as the season and congenital defects. The prevalence of infectious disease in a community affects nutritional status adversely, and poor nutritional status leads to an increased vulnerability to infection. Together with this vicious cycle it seems that malnutrition in infancy in a disadvantaged community can lead to minimal mental deficit, thereby maintaining the disadvantage already present.

Clearly the improvement of standard of living alone will do much to improve nutritional status, in part independently of dietary change. Improved nutritional status is accompanied by a reduction of health risk of almost every type and probably by a maximization of potential mental ability.

References

Alberman, E. D., Pharoah, P. O. D and Chamberlain, G. (1977) Smoking and the fetus. *Lancet,* 36–7 (letter).

Baird, D. (1977) Epidemiologic patterns over time. *In* "The Epidemiology of Prematurity", (Reed, D. M. and Stanley, F. J., eds), pp. 5–15. Urban and Schwarzenberg. Baltimore–Munich.

Baird, D. and Thomson, A. (1969). "Perinatal Problems", (Butler, N. R. and Alberman, E., eds), p. 24. E. and S. Livingstone, Edinburgh and London.

Bakketeig, L. S. and Hoffman, H. J. (1979) Perinatal mortality by birth order within cohorts based on sibship size. *British Medical Journal,* 2, 693–6.

Butler, N. R. and Alberman, E. D. (1969) "Perinatal Problems". Livingstone, Edinburgh and London.

Chamberlain, R., Chamberlain, G., Howlett, B. and Claireaux, A. (1975) "British Births 1970: Vol 1, First Week of Life". Heinemann Medical, London.

Davie, R., Butler, N. and Goldstein, H. (1972). "From Birth to Seven", p. 82. Longman, in association with the National Children's Bureau, London.

Dobbing, J. (1976) Vulnerable periods in brain growth. *In* "The Biology of Human Fetal Growth", (Roberts, D. F., and Thomson, A. M., eds). Taylor and Francis, London.

Eveleth, P. B. (1978) Population differences in growth: environmental and genetic factors. *In* "Human Growth", (Faulkner, F. and Tanner, J. M., eds) Part 3, p. 376. Balliere Tindall, London.

Eveleth, P. B. and Tanner, J. M. (1976) "Worldwide Variation in Human Growth". Cambridge University Press, London.

Falkner, F. and Tanner, J. M. (1978) "Human Growth". Balliere Tindall, London.

Garn, S. M., Shaw, H. A. and McCabe, K. D. (1977) Effects of socio-economic status and race on weight-defined and gestational prematurity in the United States. *In* "The Epidemiology of Prematurity", (Reed, D. H. and Stanley, F. J. L., eds), pp. 127–43. Urban and Schwarzenberg, Baltimore–Munich.

Garn, S. M. and Bailey, S. M., (1978) The genetics of maturational processes. *In* "Human Growth, I", (Falkner, F. and Tanner, J. M., eds), pp. 307–30. Balliere Tindall, London.

Gruenwald, P., Funakawa, H., Mitaui, S., Nishimura, T. and Takenchi, S. (1967) Influence of environmental factors on foetal growth in man. *Lancet,* i, 1026–8.

Kagan, A., Harris, B. R., Winkelstein, W., Johnson, K. G., Kato, H., Syme,

S. L., Rhoads, G. G., Gay, M. L., Nachaman, M. Z., Hamilton, H. B. and Tillotson, J. (1974) Epidemiologic studies of coronary heart disease and stroke in Japanese men living in Japan, Hawaii and California: demographic, physical, dietary and biochemical characteristics. *Journal of Chronic Diseases,* **974,** 345–64.

Kline, J., Stein, Z. A., Susser, M. and Warburton, D. (1977) Smoking: a risk factor for spontaneous abortion. *New England Journal of Medicine,* **297,** 793–6.

Lechtig, A., Delgado, H., Lasky, R. E. *et al.* (1975) Maternal nutrition and fetal growth in developing societies. *American Journal of Diseases of Children,* **129,** 434–7.

Lindgren, G. (1976) Height, weight and menarche in Swedish urban school children in relation to socio-economic and regional factors. *Annals of Human Biology,* **3,** 510–28.

MacDonald, A. (1964) "Children of Very Low Birthweight". Medical Education and Information Unit, in Association with William Heinemann Medical, London.

Mallett, R. and Knox, G. (1979) Standardised perinatal ratios, technique, utility and interpretation. *Community Medicine,* **1,** 6–13.

Metcoff, J. (1978) Association of fetal growth with maternal nutrition. *In* "Human Growth, I", (Falkner, F. and Tanner, J. M., eds), pp. 415–60. Balliere Tindall, London.

Renwick, J. H. (1972) Anencephaly and spina bifida are usually preventable by avoidance of a specific unidentified substance present in certain potato tubers. *British Journal of Preventative and Social Medicine,* **26,** 67–88.

Rush, D. (1975) Maternal nutrition during pregnancy in industrialised societies. *American Journal of Diseases of Children,* **129,** 430.

Smithells, R. W., Sheppard, S., Schorah, C. J., Seller, M. J., Nevin, N. C., Harris, R., Read, A. P. and Fielding, D. W. (1980) Possible prevention of neural tube defects by periconceptional vitamin supplementation. *Lancet,* **i,** 339–40.

Stein, Z., Susser, M., Saenger, G. and Marolla, F. (1975) "Famine and Human Development. The Dutch Hunger Winter of 1944/45". Oxford University Press, New York.

Susser, M. and Stein, Z. (1977) Prenatal nutrition and subsequent development. *In* The Epidemiology of Prematurity", (Reed, D. M. and Stanley, F. J. L., eds), pp. 177–91. Urban and Schwarzenberg, Baltimore–Munich.

Tanner, J. M. (1978) "Foetus into Man. Physical Growth from Conception to Maturity", pp. 150–128, 149. Open Books Publishing.

Thomson, A. M. (1959) Diet in pregnancy. 3. Diet in relation to the course and outcome of pregnancy. *British Journal of Nutrition,* **13,** 509–25.

Widdowson, E. M. (1951) Mental contentment and physical growth. *Lancet,* **i,** 1316–18.

World Health Organisation (1978) "World Health Organisation Study on Social and Biological Effects on Perinatal Mortality". Geneva.

Nutrition of Schoolchildren

A. E. Bender

Department of Food Science and Nutrition,
Queen Elizabeth College, London

The nutrition of the child calls for special attention since shortages to which an adult might be able to adapt without any ill-effects may hinder growth and development. A child has greater nutrient requirements in proportion to total energy intake than an adult, so the diet has to be "better"—a problem that is compounded by the possibility of children consuming inordinate amounts of sugary and "junk" foods and so effectively reducing the nutrient density of their diet.

If such foods are additional to an adequate diet the result might be obesity or the consumer might simply burn off the surplus. If they replace normal foods then they may reduce the intake of essential nutrients, but the extras would have to be very considerable in terms of "empty calories" to be effective in diluting an adequate diet. For example, 125 g of sweets supplying, say, 500 kcal, would reduce the nutrient density of a 2000 kcal diet by 25%. (In our survey of nearly 5000 children we did not observe any who regularly consumed such amounts (B∍nder *et al.,* 1977).)

Undernourished?

The clinical description that has been used to diagnose mild malnutrition—small for age, of poor muscular development, poor muscle tone, thin, pale, with little desire for exercise—is vague, subjective and difficult to interpret. Indeed, a difference in the incidence of malnutrition between England and Wales at 0·68%, and Scotland at 1·7%, was described as being "merely a reflection of different standards" (Berry and Hollingsworth, 1963).

Growth is used as the criterion in most investigations and two traditional and well-established observations have led to the belief that maximum growth rates are not only the index but the goal of good nutrition. Certainly inadequate nutrition leads to poor growth; equally maximum growth rates require an adequate supply of energy and nutrients. Consequently we tend to regard fast growth as an index of good health. In many species restriction of growth leads to a longer life-span but it is not know whether this applies to man.

The problems of human nutrition in general and child nutrition in particular are illustrated by the unexplained ability of many people in developing countries to subsist and even to lactate on energy intakes around half of the amount that we consider necessary; the tallness and apparent fitness of may people in certain areas known to be severely short of food emphasizes the problem. Whether or not this adaptation, since this is the likely explanation, is long-term starting from shortages in childhood is not known, but it does make us wonder whether our "excellent diets" are the best in the long run.

However, until we know better we must continue to feed sufficient to permit full mental and physical development at as fast a rate as is compatible with health and environmental and social conditions.

Shortness of stature can be caused by a variety of factors including medical conditions, interruption of sleep, small birthweight and environmental conditions but is usually included among nutritional indices. It is, in fact, the only practical index since nutritional deficiencies in this country are most unlikely to be sufficiently severe to cause clinical or even biochemical changes. The only clinical deficiencies reported are rickets in certain sections of the population and anaemia, which is more common but open to several interpretations.

With such difficulties in detecting mild undernutrition the only practical procedure is to try to ensure a "good" diet. Boyd Orr (1937) defined optimum nutrition as that state of nutrition which is not susceptible to improvement by the addition of any dietary supplement. This is more difficult to ascertain. Since individual variation in nutrient requirements is so great it is not possible to define a "good" diet for an individual child so we can only attempt to feed at the levels of nutrient intakes found necessary at the highest end of the scale, i.e. to use the recommended daily amounts (RDAs) of nutrients found to be necessary to ensure that even those with the highest needs are adequately nourished. We are thus always guilty of using RDAs for a purpose for which they are not intended, namely to plan the diet of the individual. If we do not do this then we cannot be sure that any individual's diet is adequate. However, for growing children we try to find support from growth rates.

School milk

In the 1920s there was malnutrition among many children in Great Britain and the classical work of Mann (1926), "Diets for boys during the school age", demonstrated the beneficial effects of supplementing the diet with 1 pint (570 ml) of milk as measured by height and weight increases.

A group of schoolboys 7–11 years of age gained 7 lb in weight and 2·6 inches in height in the first year, compared with 3·9 lb and 1·8 inches in controls. The differences were maintained over three years of observation.

The lesser though still marked effects of providing butter as a supplement indicated either a shortage of energy or vitamin A or both in the normal diets. The sickness rate was also reduced in the supplemented group.

About 10 years later milk was made available for schoolchildren to purchase at a halfpenny for one-third of a pint morning and afternoon.

In 1940 one-third of a pint was provided free for young children and in 1944 this was extended to all schoolchildren. It had been intended to provide ⅔ pint but there was not enough available.

Indeed in 1957 the Cohen Report recommended the discontinuation of welfare orange juice after the age of 2 years since the diet was considered to be adequate in vitamin C at least (Cohen, 1957).

In 1968 free milk was withdrawn from secondary schoolchildren; from 1971 it was provided free only to children under 7 except on the advice of a Medical Officer of Health. In 1971 milk ceased to be available free for expectant mothers and young children except for those in needy families.

The 1968 change was economic rather than nutritional in origin and when it was put into effect without consulting the advisory committees of the Department of Health it was widely feared that this would, or might, be detrimental to the health of children. When it was pointed out by some that one-third of a pint (190 ml) could make very little contribution to the diet it was countered that it might be of significance to a minority of poorly fed children.

Of course there were political as well as nutritional overtones. As an editorial in the Lancet put it a few years later (Lancet, 1973) "the Government's decision...met with a good deal of anger and resentment.... Indeed, so loud were some bellows of rage heard in the House of Commons that one might have been forgiven for thinking that the cows providing this milk were sacred."

In the event it does not seem to have resulted in any detectable change. Several investigations have been carried out to seek possible effects of the withdrawal of milk. It was not possible in most parts of the country to compare children before and after the change—indeed that was the main complaint from nutritionists in 1968, namely, that the possible effects should have been examined before withdrawing the milk.

Baker, Elwood and others (1978, 1980) surveyed 7- to 8-year-old children in the lowest socio-economic group—presumably those at greatest risk. A group of children who received free school meals and came from families of four or more children were provided with 190 ml milk daily for 2 years and compared with 3500 controls. There were no significant differences. (After 21·5 months the supplemented group were 3% taller (2·93 mm, $P < 0·05$) and 130 g heavier ($P < 0·05$) and the authors regard so small a difference as being of no import.)

In a longitudinal survey (using the National Study of Health and Growth) of 6- to 7-year-old children in 28 areas in 1972−3, using height as the index, Cook *et al.* (1979), also concluded that there was no difference. Scottish girls who had free milk in 1972 and 1973 were significantly taller (5 mm) than controls but Scottish boys were not. English boys were taller than controls but not girls. There was no consistency in growth over one-year periods. Moreover Scottish girls with the greatest height gain were actually consuming only one-sixth of a pint more milk in the whole diet than their controls. It was concluded that the observed differences were chance findings.

However, Reed (1978) complained that failure to stimulate growth with a dietary supplement was not evidence of failure of benefit. In particular deposition of extra calcium, detectable by X ray, might, later in life, reduce bone loss in menopausal women (osteoporosis), and he suggested that it would (might?) be of benefit to provide extra calcium during the time of bone growth.

In most countries of the world there is still a difference in heights of children of different socio-economic groups. Rona *et al.* (1979) examined 10,000 children in 28 areas of England and Scotland. Those receiving free school meals, i.e. from poorer families, were significantly shorter than both other children taking school meals and children taking other types of mid-day meals. (Figures were 0·25 standard deviation score (SDS) shorter in England; 0·5 SDS in Scotland, and 0·8 SDS in social class V in Scotland: standard deviation score is 5−7 cm). The authors concluded that a large proportion of those children receiving free school meals were of lower nutritional status than others and that withdrawal of such meals might well prejudice their future development.

School meals

School meals date from 1864 when the Destitute Children's Dinner Society was founded in response to the great need of poorly fed children in the crowded cities. The poor state revealed by the examination of conscripts for the Boer War in 1901 led to an Act of Parliament in 1906 permitting local authorities to provide free meals for certain pupils. This was slowly expanded until it covered one quarter of a million children in 1939. This number rapidly expanded during the Second World War and reached 2·25 million children by 1946 and 5·3 million in 1973. This meant that two-thirds of all children were receiving the meal.

As well as providing food the aim of school meals was to introduce children to a wider variety of foods than they might obtain at home and to inculcate social manners by eating in a group. Nutritional guidelines were laid down in 1966 by the Department of Education and Science (DES, 1966).

The average meal was intended to supply one-third of the day's needs for energy (880 kcal, 3·7 MJ) and one-half of the protein (29 g). However, as stated in that publication these figures will vary with the size of portions served to children of different age and sex. It was not clear whether this referred to the food purchased or served.

The greater problem of portion size arises from the failure to realize that children's energy requirements appear to vary over a two- or three-fold range so that a meal inadequate for one might be far too much for another. It is not even clear whether or not the child's appetite is an adequate guide to his energy needs but this must be assumed. The sizes of portions vary enormously in different schools and the methods of allowing for needs or appetite or that day's particular wants of the individual child vary equally. Portion variation was shown in a marked fashion in the survey of Bender *et al.* (1972). The average of 20 meals eaten on one day in one school was 1340 kcal, and in another, catering for the same senior age group, was 640 kcal. Equally wide was the range of meal size in infant/junior schools, varying from an average of 340 kcal in one school to 700 kcal in another. (Plate waste was similar in most schools and bore no relation to the size of the meal served.)

It is hardly likely that the *average* energy requirements of children of similar ages differ so widely so some children must have been provided with less food than they needed. This was borne out in examining methods of taking care of appetite differences. In some schools, both in that and our later survey, children were asked whether they wanted a small, medium or large portion (although the answer was often ignored and all received the same); others offered "seconds" if food was left. Many of those who asked for "seconds" could not be given any so it would seem that some were not getting as much as they wanted.

Taking the target as the recommended dietary amount for children of each age group, infant schools achieved 70% of the energy and 57% of the protein target; infant/junior schools achieved 69% of energy and 60% of

Table I

Average meal *eaten* (median and range) in schools in Essex Survey on single occasion (average of 20 meals per school). Energy and protein calculated from weighed portions (Bender et al., 1972).

Type of school	Number of schools	Energy (kcal)			Protein (g)		
		Target[a]	Eaten median (range)	Per cent target	Target[a]	Eaten median (range)	Per cent target
Infant	8	600	420 (360—640)	70	23	13 (10—16)	57
Infant/junior	18	700	480 (330—790)	69	25	15 (11—30)	60
Junior	12	750	475 (280—660)	63	29	16 (8—26)	55
Senior	10	870	650 (420—1340)	75	33	20 (11—31)	61

[a]Targets are one-third RDA for children in middle of age range of each type of school.

Table II

Average meal *served* in schools in Brent survey over 5 days. Energy and protein as calculated from weighed portions (Bender et al., 1977).

Type of school	Number of schools	Age group (years)	No. of pupils	Energy			Protein		
				Served (MJ)	Per cent target[a]	Plate waste (MJ)	Served (g)	Per cent target[a]	Plate waste (g)
Infant	2	5—7	525	1·64	65	0·19	14·5	76	1·9
Infant/Junior	2	5—11	760	2·21	76	0·39	16·9	77	3·3
Junior	4	7—11	1544	2·19	70	0·13	17·3	74	1·4
Middle	2	11—15	821	3·06	86	0·28	21·5	81	2·5
Senior	2	15—18+	1144	3·51	95	0·23	24·1	86	1·6

[a]Target one-third RDA energy, 42% protein, according to age.

protein target; junior schools achieved 63% of energy and 55% of protein targets; senior schools achieved 75% of energy and 61% of protein targets (Table I). These were the median figures for the amount eaten in schools in each group.

In 1975 the DES guidelines were modified—"children in each age group should be served on the plate at minimum one third of the recommended daily intake of energy and one third to one half of the RDI for protein." (DES, 1975). This would not differ much from the earlier amounts if the wording in the 1966 guidelines, "with due allowance for age" was interpreted by reference to tables of RDI. For senior pupils this would be 3·69 MJ (885 kcal) and 28 g protein compared with the earlier amounts stated as being 880 kcal and 29 g protein.

Our second survey (Bender *et al.*, 1977) examined the meals of 4794 pupils daily for five days. The previous survey had been cross-sectional on a larger number of schools visited on a single occasion. Total food purchased, with allowance for measured kitchen waste, revealed food available per head. This was cross-checked by weighing 20 meals as served on the plate—the figures did agree. As before, plate waste was measured to ascertain food eaten.

Using the targets of one-third of RDI energy for each age group and 42% protein the target achievements were as follows: (a) infants 65% energy, 76% protein; (b) infant/junior 76% and 77%, respectively; (c) junior 70% and 74%; (d) middle, 86% and 81%; (e) senior 95% and 86% (Table II). These were the amounts offered on the plate and waste reduced the amount eaten by approximately 10% on average.

These figures were similar to our earlier survey (Bender *et al.*, 1972) and to those of Essex-Cater and Robert-Sargeant (1975), but lower than those found by Cook *et al.* (1975).

A number of problems are raised that have not been discussed previously. Firstly, are the targets correct? RDAs for nutrients other than protein are based on average needs plus 2 standard deviations (SDs) to take care of the needs of those at the highest end of the scale. If the distribution curve of nutrient consumption matched that of nutrient requirements then there would be no need to add 2 SD to average requirements. It is to ensure that those with highest needs obtain them that the average for all diets in any group are set at the high figures. This problem of RDA is a fundamental one. RDA for energy, however, does not include the surplus but is supposed to be the average of what is eaten. Many of those working in the field of energy intake would argue that it is past time when such figures were re-examined—average intakes in so many surveys are well below these figures. Similarly, protein RDAs in Great Britain are set at 10% of the energy intake (for reasons of palatability and the fact that protein foods carry many other nutrients)—a figure that is about double physiological needs. So is it a matter of any nutritional significance if the average intakes of children fall below these rather artificial figures and was the nutritional advisory committee at fault in attempting to get 42% of the protein into 33% of the energy in the school meal?

Secondly, far too little attention has been paid to the very large differences in the needs, wants and appetites of different individual children.

Thirdly, since many requesting second helpings of the school dinner could not be supplied were some children going hungry?

Fourthly, with the current changes from the traditional meals to snacks, cafeteria systems, convenience foods, ready-made meals and sandwich meals, should local authorities be aiming at the original targets, those amounts that the children actually received or should targets be reconsidered?

An example of the lack of clarity is the experiment offering textured vegetable protein (TVP) in place of meat at school meals in Leeds (Glew, personal communication). The waste on the plate was somewhat greater than usual and might be considered due to the relative unattractiveness of TVP, but it was not clear whether the children had been offered the small amount that they were used to being offered as meat, or the target amount suggested in the DES circulars, or larger quantities than usual.

The reasons for the shortfall in the size of the meals, whether the target was correct or not, are manifold (Bender *et al.*, 1977).

a) The amounts of food purchased were usually insufficient to meet the targets even before allowing for kitchen waste.

b) Lack of catering expertise resulted in buying the cheapest cuts of meat, trimming off unwanted fat and gristle in the kitchen and finishing up with not-so-cheap meat on the plate. No one appears to have considered the cost-benefit of buying a "better" cut of meat.

c) Acceptance of delivery of poor quality vegetables resulted in considerable quantities of inedible matter being trimmed off with consequent reduction in amounts available and increase in cost per portion.

d) Wastage in the kitchen, apart from normal kitchen waste, was very considerable. In some schools in order to be certain that enough food was left for later servings quite small portions were given and as a result food was left over at the end of the meal and *thrown away*. In another area the reverse was true of meat since the later feeders were given only vegetables and no meat.

e) Portion control, surely top priority in catering teaching, was almost completely ignored and there was often 100% difference in the size of portions served to adjacent plates intended to be the same.

f) There was often a complete lack of liaison between the advisor in the office and the staff in the kitchen, with consequent lack of instruction and guidance.

g) Some of the most bizarre cooking methods were employed. For example, in some schools, potatoes were peeled the day before and left soaking in water overnight since "there was no time to peel them before lunch." On being asked how this problem was overcome on Mondays the answer was that two lots were peeled on a Monday. When minced meat pie was being prepared (and this personally observed at least in one school) the minced meat was boiled for 90 minutes, the cooking water— gravy— containing the greater part, if not 100%, of the water-soluble nutrients was discarded and the "filtered" meat used.

h) There was no exchange of information and ideas between schools. If one school can provide 1340 kcal in the average meal for, presumably, the same cost as another can provide only 640 kcal it would seem that one could teach the other.

Possibly the greatest criticism of those involved in the school meals service is the complete lack of evaluation. Of the four published surveys of school meals, three were carried out by research groups, and only one of these at the instigation of the local authority; nothing was ever attempted by the responsible groups in the Department of Education and Science in the days when they were responsible for the meals. Before this statement is criticized in absolute terms, I am aware that for some part of the time the Inner London Education Authority did examine some meals—about 50 plates were examined per year.

Current problems

A major change took place from April 1980 when the Education Bill in effect released the local authorities from nutritional confines. In the era of saving money many modifications could be made in the traditional "meat-and-two-veg" type of school meal and indeed cafeteria systems with a wider choice have been in operation to some extent for some time. Alternatives are (a) snacks, (b) sandwiches and soups, (c) purchase of convenience foods to varying extents in place of meals cooked at the school, and (d) freeze-thaw systems.

Changes, where there are any, are intended to save money (meaning staff wages), improve the efficiency of organization and management, and maintain nutritional standards. The problem worrying some authorities is the maintenance of nutritional standards. They do not know where to go for advice, opinions differ in any case and the whole problem is shaded by emotional overtones of local councillors. There are headteachers as well as councillors who think that anything other than a traditional meal cannot be satisfactory and that sandwiches are an abomination. When the price of school meals has been increased in the past there has been a decrease, usually temporary, in attendance. The main alternative for children is to bring sandwiches from home and this has given rise to major arguments of principle on what appear to be extremely trivial matters such as "where will the children eat their sandwiches" and "who will clean the floor?" Are we expecting those who buy a school meal to subsidize the sandwich-bringers? Such trivia are on a par with the "problem" of avoiding indicating those children who are allowed free meals. The simple solutions have so far evaded the authorities.

There is great scope for saving money and improving the attraction of the meal from the child's point of view. Indeed some reports suggest that snack meals have proved so popular that larger numbers of children are taking the school meal. It may be necessary to distinguish between "snack meals" and "snack foods". "Snack meals" include popular dishes like beans-on-toasts, sausages, fish fingers and hamburgers, all of which can be as nutritious as any traditional meal. Judging from the portions provided in the past in those schools surveyed it is likely that such snacks will provide a greater intake of nutrients. Even sandwiches and soup will provide more than many of the meals referred to here.

"Snack foods" on the other hand tend to mean potato crisps, sweets, chocolate bars and peanuts.

With the school meal now costing up to 60 pence there is ample scope for manufactured foods to play a role in the meal, probably at less cost. It should not be difficult to buy wholesale, in bulk, manufactured foods that are attractive to children, satisfy nutritional needs and save money.

Hamburgers are very popular and much advertising play is made of the fact that they are 100% meat, or, in some products, nearly so. In fact we have examined such preparations made from less than 40% meat (with cereal and vegetables making up the rest) which contained the same amounts of protein of the same quality (as measured on experimental animals) as the "better" commercial products, with the same content of iron and of thiamin (used as indicators on nutrient content), and which were as acceptable to hospital patients as traditional dishes.

Conclusions

Despite criticisms of the traditional meals, and although several children appeared to be in need of dietary care, there was no evidence to suggest that they were at educational, nutritional or medical risk. Before we embark on further discussions relating to this emotional, political and financially heavy burden we need to find out what we are really worrying about—or indeed if there is any cause for concern.

References

Baker, I. A., Elwood, P. C., Hughes, J., Jones, M. and Sweetnan, D. M. (1978) School milk and growth in primary schoolchildren. *Lancet,* **ii,** 575.

Baker, I. A. *et al.* (1980) A randomised controlled trial of the effect of the provision of free school milk on the growth of children. *Journal of Epidemiology and Community Health,* **34,** 31−4.

Bender, A. E., Magee, P. and Nash, A. H. (1972) Survey of school meals. *British Medical Journal,* **2,** 383−5.

Bender, A. E., Harris, M. C. and Getreuer, A. (1977) Feeding of school children in a London borough. *British Medical Journal,* **1,** 757−9.

Berry, W. T. C. and Hollingsworth, D. F. (1963) *Proceedings of the Nutrition Society,* **22,** 48.

Essex-Cater, A. and Robert-Sargeant, S. (1975) *Health and Social Services Journal,* **85,** 758.

Cohen, H. (1957) "Report of the Joint Sub-Committee on Welfare Foods". HMSO, London.

Cook, J., Altman, D. G., Jacoby, A., Holland, W. W. and Elliot, A. (1975) School meals and nutrition of schoolchildren. *British Journal of Preventative and Social Medicine,* **29,** 182−9.

Cook, J., Irwig, L. M., Chinn, S., Altman, D. G. and Florey, C. du V. (1979) The influence of availability of free school milk in England and Scotland. *Journal of Epidemiology and Community Health,* **33,** 171.

Department of Education and Science (1966). "The Nutritional Standard of School Dinners", Circular 3/66. HMSO, London.

Department of Education and Science (1975) "Nutrition in Schools". HMSO, London.

Lancet (1973) Editorial: Free milk from the sacred cow. *Lancet,* **ii,** 183.

Mann, H. C. C. (1926) "Diets for Boys During the School Age". Medical Research Council Report No. 105. HMSO, London.

Orr, J. B. (1937) "Health, Food and Income", 2nd edn, p. 7. Macmillan, London.

Reed, F. B. (1978) School milk and growth in schoolchildren. *Lancet,* **ii,** 675−6.

Rona, R. J., Chinn, S. and Smith, A. M. (1979) *Lancet,* **ii,** 534.

Socio-economic Influences of Nutrient Intake in Children

M. Nelson and A. A. Paul

Medical Research Council,
Dunn Nutrition Unit, Cambridge

One of the major determinants of growth and health in children is social class. The theme "preventive nutrition" suggests that we should be investigating whether these social class differences in development are dietary in origin, or if they are due to non-nutritional environmental influences. To do this, we must first look at social class differences in health, growth and diet, and then consider the results of studies in which dietary intervention has been used in an attempt to improve the children's development.

Morris (1979) has shown that the standardized mortality ratio for all causes of death in men in social class (SC) V is almost twice that for SC I, while there is a three-fold difference in the post-neonatal death rate per 1000 live births between the lowest and highest social classes (Table I). Similarly, the rate of chronic sickness amongst children is highest in SC V. Nelson and Naismith (1979) have also reported that rates for reduction in normal levels of activity due to illness, for visits to doctors, and for treatment of chronic complaints were two or three times higher amongst poor children than amongst children in the general population.

Table I

Health indices by social class (from Morris, 1979).

	Social class	
	I	V
Standardized mortality ratio (all causes, men 15—64 years)	77	137
Infant mortality (post natal deaths per 1000 live births)	2·8	8·6
Chronic sickness (children 0—14 years, rates per 1000)	92	123

Growth is also correlated with social class. In the National Child Development Study (Goldstein, 1971), 7-year-olds from SC I were between 2 and 3 cm taller than those from SC V. More recently, a study was carried out in Wales in which the proportion of children receiving free school meals was used as an index of environmental quality in different schools (Baker *et al.*, 1979). In the schools where up to 9% of the children were receiving free school meals, 8-year-old children from SC IV and V were on average 2 cm shorter than SC I and II 8-year-olds, but where 30% or more of the children were receiving free school meals, SC IV and V children were on average 4 cm shorter than SC I and II children (Table II). Similar findings have been reported for children living in England and Scotland (Rona *et al.*, 1979).

Table II

Height (cm) of 8-year-old Welsh children by social class and type of school; based on proportion of children receiving free school meals (from Baker *et al.*, 1979).

Percent of children	Height (cm)	
receiving free school meals:	0–9%	30% or more
Social class		
I + II	130	130
III manual	129	128
IV + V	128	126

Whereas all studies of child growth in Britain have reported the average height in SC I children to be greater than that of children in SC V, the relationship between weight or obesity and social class is not so clear cut. Some authors (Whitelaw, 1971; Stunkard *et al.*, 1972; Silverstone, 1974) have reported higher weights and skinfold thicknesses in lower social class children, while others (Nelson and Naismith, 1979; Durnin *et al.*, 1974; Topp *et al.*, 1970) have reported lower weights and skinfold thicknesses in the lower social classes.

Changes in nutrient intake since 1938

It is important to look first at the changes in nutrient intake which have taken place during the last 40 years, a period of generally increasing affluence and diminishing levels of activity. The energy intakes of 3-year-olds and of 14-year-old boys and girls have been plotted in Fig. 1 using

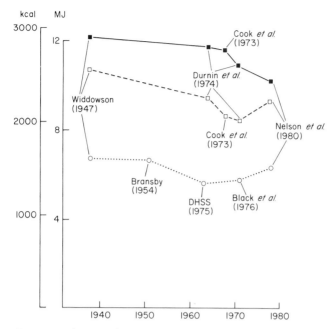

Figure 1 Energy intakes per day (expressed as kcal and MJ) in children from 1938 to 1978. ■-■ Males, 14 years;□-□females, 14 years;O-O males and females, 3 years.

results from studies spanning 1938 to 1978. The 1938 results were based on the intakes of middle-class children (Widdowson, 1947), while the later studies covered children from a wider range of socio-economic background (Durnin *et al.*, 1974; Cook *et al.*, 1973; Bransby and Fothergill, 1954; Department of Health and Social Security, 1975; Black *et al.*, 1976; Nelson *et al.*, 1980).

It can be seen clearly that energy intakes have declined in all three groups, particularly amongst 14-year-old boys. The slight upward trend in energy intakes amongst 14-year-old girls and 3-year-olds in 1978 is probably due to sampling limitations in the 1978 survey (Nelson *et al.*, 1980). The decline in the intakes of energy is also reflected in results from the National Food Survey (Ministry of Food, 1954; Ministry of Agriculture, Fisheries and Food, 1955–80) in which the average energy intake per person per day in households with 2 adults and 2 children has fallen by 9·6% from 2256 kcal in 1952 to 2042 kcal in 1978. During this same period the recommended intakes for energy were also substantially reduced, by as much as 30% in the case of 16-year-old girls (British Medical Association, 1950; Department of Health and Social Security, 1979).

Table III

Diet quality: nutrient intakes of children per 1000 kcal.

	1938 (Widdowson, 1947)	1978 (Nelson *et al.*, 1980)
Protein (g)	29·2	30·4
Calcium (mg)	344	482
Iron (mg)	5·1	4·9
Thiamin (mg)	0·35	0·58
Vitamin C (mg)	24	22

Surprisingly, there has been little change in the quality of the diet over this period. Intakes of protein, iron, and vitamin C per 1000 kcal in 1978 were virtually the same as they were in 1938 (Table III). Only for calcium and thiamin have there been any appreciable increases. The increase in calcium intake is not attributable to milk consumption which, if anything, appears to have declined slightly over the years, from 5·4 pints per child per week in 1938 (Widdowson, 1947) to 4·3 pints per child per week in 1977 (Ministry of Agriculture, Fisheries and Food, 1955–80). The fortification of flour with calcium and the increase in cheese consumption does account for most of the change, however. The increase in thiamin per 1000 kcal is again attributable to the fortification of flour, and also to improvements in the analytical data available in the tables of food composition (Paul and Southgate, 1978) on which the most recent estimates of nutrient intake are based. In fact, as energy intakes have declined, fortification appears to have played an increasingly important role in maintaining adequate intakes. The range of foods fortified today is much wider than 40 years ago, and yet the diet quality appears to have changed very little.

The fat in the average diet in 1978 contributed 39% of the dietary energy compared with 37% in the middle-class diets in 1938, as shown in Table IV. This change has been offset by a corresponding reduction in the contribution of carbohydrate to energy intake, the energy from protein having remained unchanged.

Table IV

Per cent of dietary energy from protein fat and carbohydrate in children's diets.

	1938 (Widdowson, 1947)	1978 (Nelson *et al.*, 1980)
Protein	12	12
Fat	37	39
Carbohydrate	51	49

Social class differences in diet

Prior to the Second World War, there were large differences between the more adequate diets of the middle class and the diets of poorer families. Widdowson (1947) recorded the intakes of 38 children whose fathers were unemployed members of the "artisan" class, the semi-skilled and unskilled workers. The energy intakes of these children up to age 9 years were, surprisingly, only slightly lower than the average middle-class intakes, and from 10 to 13 years of age the energy intakes in the two groups were similar. In contrast, the intakes of calcium, iron, and other nutrients in the poorer children were almost all below the average middle-class intakes. The girls especially had very low intakes of all nutrients.

In their national study of diet and health in pre-war Britain, the Rowett Research Institute (1955) divided families into six food expenditure groups, and expressed the average family intakes as a percentage of the British Medical Association (1950) standards. For energy, the highest food expenditure group had intakes of 125% of the standard, while the lowest group had intakes only 70% of the standard, a difference of 55% of the standard between the two groups. Differences between the highest and lowest group intakes of protein, calcium, and vitamin A were 65%, 80% and 60% of the standard respectively. Although the clinical examination of the poorest-fed group revealed no frank deficiency disease, the growth and health of these children was much poorer than that of their better-fed contemporaries. Some of the nutritional limitations to the poorest children's development were overcome through a food intervention study. A food supplement which included soup, milk, cheese, wheat-germ, marmite, halibut liver oil capsules and oranges was given to an experimental group whose subsequent development was shown to be superior to that of the unsupplemented controls. The greatest degree of improvement was observed in the children from the very poorest families.

During and after the war, the nutritional picture changed dramatically. By 1943, the differences in the adequacy of diet (expressed as a percentage of the League of Nations standards) between the highest and lowest food expenditure groups had shrunk to less than 26% for energy, protein, calcium, iron and thiamin, and to less than 40% for vitamins A and C (Wagner and Whitelaw, 1945). More recent studies conducted between 1963 and 1971 have shown only small and inconsistent differences in intakes between social classes. Average energy, calcium, and iron intakes of pre-school children from SC IV and V were in fact greater than the average intakes of these nutrients amongst SC I and II children of the same age (Department of Health and Social Security, 1975). In Durnin's study of 14-year-old children in Glasgow (Durnin *et al.,* 1974), the intakes of these same three nutrients were 10–15% lower in boys from the lowest social class compared with the intakes of boys from the highest social class, while the lowest social class girls had lower intakes of calcium, but higher intakes of energy and iron compared with the highest social class girls.

In our Cambridge study (Nelson *et al.*, 1980), children's intakes did not vary consistently by social class. The children's energy and iron intakes expressed as a percentage of the RDA (DHSS, 1979) were fairly uniform by social class (Figs 2 and 3), with the exception of energy intakes in males

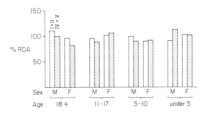

Figure 2   Energy intakes in adults and children in 66 Cambridge families, expressed as a percentage of RDA (DHSS, 1979), by sex, age-group, and social class:☐I + II;▨IV + V (from Nelson *et al.*, 1980).

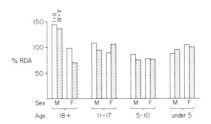

Figure 3   Iron intakes in adults and children in 66 Cambridge families, expressed as a percentage of RDA (DHSS, 1979), by sex, age-group, and social class:☐I + II;▨IV + V (from Nelson *et al.*, 1980).

under 5 years old, in which a certain amount of overfeeding appeared to be taking place in the social class IV and V families. Iron intakes appeared to be more dependent on age than on social class. This may simply be a reflection of differences in the RDA in relation to intake at different ages, and is not necessarily a true measure of the relative adequacy of the diet in the different age groups. Only dietary fibre intakes showed consistent social class trends, being higher in SC I and II children than in SC IV and V children in all but one age/sex group (Fig. 4).

Two features of the adults' intakes are worth noting (Figs 2, 3 and 4).

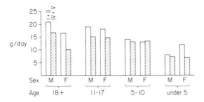

Figure 4 Fibre intakes in adults and children in 66 Cambridge families, grams per day, by sex, age group, and social class:☐I + II;▨IV + V (from Nelson *et al.*, 1980).

First, there was a consistent tendency in both men and women for the higher social class individuals to have higher nutrient intakes than those from the lower social classes. Second, men's iron intakes expressed as a percentage of the RDA (DHSS, 1979) were much greater than for any other age/sex group. It appeared that the men were receiving far more than their "fair share" of iron, in terms of the RDA, and that this was at the expense of women and girls between 5 and 10 years of age in particular. It is interesting that a similar pattern of intake in the different age/sex groups appeared in both the higher and lower social classes, suggesting that one of the factors regulating children's intakes may be a socially determined pattern of food and nutrient distribution within the family which is not bounded by social class.

Does this mean that, with the exception of dietary fibre, there are no longer any significant social-class trends in children's nutrient intake, and that the observed social class differences in growth and health are attributable only to non-nutritional environmental factors? Or does it mean that poor children in fact need more food and a better diet than their richer contemporaries, in order to help them overcome some of the stresses imposed by a poor environment? The fact that nutrient intakes in different social classes are now comparable does not automatically imply that the nutritional value of the diet is everywhere the same.

In a comparison of children's diets in different social classes in Newcastle and London (Nelson, 1980) it was observed that apparently similar diets were associated with quite different patterns of growth in children from the London manual and the Newcastle non-manual workers' families (Table V). The proportion of children falling below the 25th percentile for height was 32% in the London manual group compared with only 15% in the Newcastle non-manual group. Significantly, where intakes of nutrients in the Newcastle manual group were higher than in the London manual group, only 21% of the children were below the 25th percentile for height. It appears that in the Newcastle manual group the better diet afforded some degree of protection against environmental influences which were growth

Table V

Mean nutrient intakes expressed as a percentage of the Recommended Daily Amount and proportion of children falling at or below the 25th percentile for height (from Nelson, 1980).

Nutrient	London manual	Newcastle non-manual	Newcastle manual
Energy	86	86	103
Protein	116	111	120
Iron	98	82	94
Thiamin	114	113	122
Proportion of children ⩽ 25th percentile for height (%)	32	15	21

limiting. THUS, THE DIETS OF CHILDREN FROM LOWER SOCIAL CLASSES MAY NEED TO BE NOT SIMPLY AS GOOD AS THE DIETS OF CHILDREN FROM HIGHER SOCIAL CLASSES, BUT ACTUALLY BETTER THAN THE HIGHER SOCIAL CLASS DIETS IN ORDER TO CONFER THE SAME NUTRITIONAL BENEFITS. The corollary of this conclusion is that where children from lower social classes have poor nutrient intakes, health and growth are likely to be much worse than in higher social class children with similarly poor diets.

Intervention studies and preventive nutrition

There have been no controlled nutrition intervention studies in the UK in the last 40 years to determine whether or not a better diet for children from lower social class, or poor, families would improve their health and development. I think there have been two main reasons for this. The first is that since the war, school dinners were intended to make good any shortfall in nutrient intake amongst poor children. School dinners are, in a sense, a supplement to the diets of poor children in that they are free to those who cannot afford them. Secondly, since the 1960s, studies comparing children's intakes by social class have shown only small differences, and it has therefore been assumed that there are no further improvements to be made to the diets of poor children.

Results from the Headstart Program in the USA suggest that there is still room for improvement. It is estimated that about 30% of the poorest children have achieved better health and educational development through improvements in their diets (Lewin, 1977). Studies in London (Nelson and Naismith, 1979) and Bristol (Davis *et al.,* 1978) suggest that there are substantial numbers of poor children from broken or overcrowded homes or from families on long-term Supplementary Benefit who would benefit from a nutrition intervention programme. This is the only way in which to test whether or not we have reached the limits of nutritional improvements which would be of specific benefit to children in the lower social class.

References

Baker, I. A., Elwood, P. C. and Sweetnam, P. M. (1979) Free school meals and height of Welsh schoolchildren. *Lancet,* **ii,** 692.

Black, A. E., Billewicz, W. Z. and Thomson, A. M. (1976) The diets of pre-school children in Newcastle-upon-Tyne 1968–71. *Brit. J. Nutr.,* **35,** 105–13.

Bransby, E. R. and Fothergill, J. E. (1954) The diets of young children. *Brit. J. Nutr.,* **8,** 195–204.

British Medical Association (1950) "Report of the Committee on Nutrition". BMA, London.

Cook, J., Altman, D. G., Moore, D. M. C., Topp, S. G., Holland, W. W. and Elliot, A. (1973) A survey of the nutritional status of schoolchildren. Relation between nutrient intake and socio-economic factors. *Brit. J. Prev. Soc. Med.,* **27,** 91–9.

Davis, D. R., Apley, J., Fill, G. and Grimaldi, C. (1978) Diet and retarded growth. *Brit. Med. J.,* **1,** 539–42.

Department of Health and Social Security (1975) "A Nutrition Survey of Pre-school Children, 1967–8", Report on Health and Social Subjects No. 10. HMSO, London.

Department of Health and Social Security (1979). "Recommended Daily Amounts of Food Energy and Nutrients for Groups of People in the United Kingdom". HMSO, London.

Durnin, J. V. G. A., Lonergan, M. E., Good, J. and Ewan, A. (1974) A cross-sectional nutritional and anthropometric study, with an interval of 7 years, on 611 young adolescent schoolchildren. *Brit. J. Nutr.,* **32,** 169–79.

Goldstein, H. (1971) Factors influencing the height of seven year old children—results from the National Child Development Study. *Hum. Biol.,* **43,** 92–111.

Lewin, R. (1977) Head-start pays off. *New Scientist,* 3 March, 508–9.

Ministry of Food (1954) "Domestic Food Consumption and Expenditure, 1952". HMSO, London.

Ministry of Agriculture, Fisheries and Food (1955–1980) "Household Food Consumption and Expenditure, 1953–1978". HMSO, London.

Morris, J. N. (1979) Social inequalities undiminished. *Lancet,* **i,** 87–90.

Nelson, M. (1980) Assessing dietary intake and its relation to growth in British children. *Proc. Nutr. Soc.,* **39,** 35–42.

Nelson, M. and Naismith, D. J. (1979) The nutritional status of poor children in

London. *J. Hum. Nutr.,***33**, 33–45.

Nelson, M., Nettleton, P. A. and Paul, A. A. (1980) Unpublished results.

Paul, A. A. and Southgate, D. A. T. (1978) "McCance and Widdowson's: The Composition of Foods", 4th edn. HMSO, London.

Rona, R. J., Chinn, S. and Smith, A. M. (1979) Height of children receiving free school meals. *Lancet,* **ii**, 534.

Rowett Research Institute (1955) "Family Diet and Health in Pre-war Britain: A Dietary and Clinical Survey". Carnegie United Kingdom Trust, Dunfermline.

Silverstone, J. T. (1974) Psychological and social factors in the pathogenesis of obesity. *In* "Obesity Symposium". Churchill Livingstone, London.

Stunkard, A., d'Aquili, E., Fox, S. and Filion, R. (1972) Influence of social class on obesity and thinness in children. *J. Am. Med. Ass.,* **221**, 579–84.

Topp, S. G., Cook, J., Holland, W. W. and Elliott, A. (1970) Influence of environmental factors on height and weight of schoolchildren. *Brit. J. Prev. Soc. Med.,* **24**, 154–62.

Wagner, G. and Whitelaw, E. (1945) "A Dietary Survey of Stoke and Salford School Children", Social Survey N.S. 47. Central Office of Information, London.

Whitelaw, A. G. L. (1971) The association of social class and sibling number with skinfold thickness in London schoolboys. *Hum. Biol.,* **43**, 414–20.

Widdowson, E. M. (1947) "A study of Individual Children's Diets", Medical Research Council Special Report Series No. 257. HMSO, London.

The Role of Clinical Evaluation in Nutritional Surveillance

Angus M. Thomson

MRC Reproduction and Growth Unit,
Newcastle upon Tyne

Nearly fifteen years ago Jelliffe (1966) noted that:

> The cheapness and relatively easy organization of nutritional assessment by means of clinical examination have sometimes led to the assumption that the method is simple, quickly mastered by the beginner, and yields results that are easy to interpret. This is not the case.

There are few sharp boundaries which distinguish the normal or adequate from the abnormal or inadequate. Some children may be thin and listless and show specific abnormalities, but is this a transient or chronic state and is it due to a defective diet or to some other cause? To quote Jelliffe again: "While a few physical signs are pathognomonic (of dietary defects)...this is not usually the case." We can seldom attribute the deplorable clinical condition of young children in developing countries to a single dietary cause such as protein deficiency. The causes are nearly always multiple and usually complex; they involve, as well as shortage and imbalance of diets, such factors as infectious disease and faulty child-rearing practices. The cause of better nutrition is not advanced by campaigns based on simple theories, such as that which McLaren (1974) described as "the great protein fiasco". Referring to the clinical diagnosis of so-called protein malnutrition, McLaren wrote that: "Most (signs) turned out to be unrelated to nutrition and the rest proved non-specific".

Nutritional surveillance implies an ability to measure the incidence of specific signs of unsatisfactory nutrition and to detect changes. Yet in the absence of clear and unequivocal signs, how does one decide what proportion of children are indeed underfed or malnourished, and find out whether the situation is improving or deteriorating?

In countries like Britain, obvious and unequivocal forms of malnutrition have practically disappeared except when they are secondary to other disease or exotic social factors. Nutritional surveillance is therefore even more difficult than it is in developing countries. I have not found any reference to malnutrition in the latest Annual Report of the Chief Medical Officer (Department of Health and Social Security, 1980). It might therefore be argued that there is no need for nutritional surveillance in Britain. Yet, in 1971, the Government decided to curtail the provision of welfare foods and school milk, presumably after deciding (correctly, as it turned out) that any adverse effect on health would be negligible. But it could not be sure, in 1971, that there would be no adverse effects, and a programme of surveillance was organized (Department of Health and Social Security, 1973, 1981). Since then, the economic climate has continued to deteriorate, and the association of poverty and malnutrition (Orr, 1937) may again become relevant to food policy. Nutritional surveillance remains necessary, not least for reassurance. The problem is, how?

Ostensibly, the aim of surveillance is to assess the nutritional state of the community. (I am not concerned in this paper with clinical surveillance of individual patients.) In practice, it is almost impossible to distinguish "nutritional status" from the "general state of health", of which nutritional status forms a part. Nutritional status may be assumed to comprise those aspects of general health which can be plausibly related to the types and amounts of food consumed by members of the community, and which may be affected for better or worse by changes in diet. Since such aspects are difficult to define in a positive way, it may sound easier to do so by excluding defects of general health which are *not* directly related to diet, e.g. accidental injuries and lung cancer. But even a policy of exclusion is not easy, because food is as fundamental to health and well-being as air, water and shelter. Nutrition is therefore relevant, directly or indirectly, to a wide range of the indicators of general levels of community health. By contrast, there are very few indicators of "nutritional status" in its traditional, specific sense. The term therefore, has little clinical or scientific value, even though it continues to be a useful phrase in general discussions.

In the rest of this paper I shall review rather briefly some of the methods of approach. These methods have changed remarkably little during the past fifty years. History shows that many ideas have been promoted only to be found wanting, and have faded away.

Health statistics

Death rates by cause are published regularly and in considerable detail in this country, but are of little direct value in nutritional surveillance. Official returns for 1978 for England and Wales show only three deaths registered as due to "avitaminosis and other nutritional deficiency" out of a total of 7881 deaths in children under one year of age.

On a more general plane, it is reasonable to suppose that a generally malnourished population will tend to have high death rates from a multitude of causes, because of lowered resistance to disease. But such a concept does not get us very far nowadays. The general rates in infants and children have fallen so low that they provide rather insensitive indicators of community health. In adults, debate continues on the extent to which death rates from such causes as cardiovascular and gastro-intestinal diseases can be attributed to over-eating, or to such dietary imbalance as insufficient fibre. At present, it would be rash to consider such death rates as specific indicators of nutritional status even if we believe that dietary changes would be beneficial.

Death is such a definite event that it has obvious advantages from the point of view of statistics. Morbidity statistics are much less reliable, although the data from Hospitals' Activity Analysis and the Hospitals' In-Patient Enquiry do give us some idea of the extent and nature of serious illness in the population. We may agree that some diseases have their roots in gluttony (including alcoholism) and that it is better to keep the bowels open by eating sufficient fibre than by recourse to aperients. But I doubt if we know enough to use statistics of "the diseases of affluence" to impose dietary change on the population by legislative or administrative action. From a historical point of view, we need more work on the extent to which changes in the prevalence of specific diseases and symptom-categories may have been influenced by changes in nutrition. For example, McKeown and Record (1962) concluded from a study of falling tuberculosis mortality during the nineteenth century that the most important factor seemed to be "a rising standard of living, of which the most significant feature was improved diet".

For the reasons already discussed, I see little advantage to be gained at present from a search for specifically "nutritional" signs and symptoms during *ad hoc* surveys of general health. This is not to deny their relevance when specific hypotheses have to be investigated, e.g. that rickets and osteomalacia occur among Asian immigrants to Britain (Department of Health and Social Security, 1980) or that hypernatraemic dehydration is occurring in unsuitably-fed infants (Department of Health and Social Security, 1974).

Biochemical indices

In theory, laboratory examination of samples of body fluids such as urine or bloods can tell us a great deal about nutritional status, and they are widely used in monitoring the health of individual patients. Their usefulness is much more limited in the nutritional surveillance of communities. Ethical difficulties arise in obtaining blood samples from apparently healthy individuals, and there are nearly always problems of interpretation.

More blood samples are taken for the diagnosis of anaemia than for any other purpose. Haematological statistics can be derived from the records of the Blood Transfusion Service, but those who go to blood donor centres can scarcely be regarded as a random sample of the population. Haematological examinations are also made routinely in most antenatal clinics. Here, however, we have the awkward fact that haemoglobin concentrations fall considerably during pregnancy in women who are manifestly healthy and well-fed. In my opinion, ignorance of this physiological fact has led to excessive diagnoses of "anaemia", and to consumption of iron pills by perfectly healthy women in large and unnecessary quantities.

Growth

The relevance of growth rates and measurements of physique to nutritional surveillance is obvious. Stock farmers use live-weight gain as a prime indicator of economic efficiency in the feeding of animals. Laboratory scientists have for long used growth rates to distinguish between the effects of different diets given to experimental animals. So it seems curious that measurements of growth and body size have not been systematically exploited in the nutritional surveillance of human populations, especially since such measurements can usually be made with considerable precision and without involving ethical difficulties.

There are, of course, problems in theory as well as in practice. Unlike farmers, doctors are interested in growth as an indicator of health rather than of economic efficiency. Bigger is not self-evidently better, and excess weight is notoriously associated with social as well as medical disabilities. Unlike laboratory animals, human beings do not live in a closely controlled environment, and many factors other than nutrition may influence growth rate and body size, for example, housing, infectious diseases and exercise. Yet the importance of the nutritional factor remains. Good growth cannot occur even in an excellent general environment unless the building materials derived from food are provided.

There is, therefore, a strong *prima facie* case that systematic anthropometric studies would be valid and useful in nutritional surveillance. But which measurements are likely to give the best returns for effort expended? Skinfold thickness is certainly relevant to obesity, and the literature describes numerous formulae based on body measurements which are allegedly specially relevant to nutrition; few stood the test of time. I think we ought to start with height and weight. Growth in height is relatively stable and may be considered to be affected by long-term nutritional influences, whereas weight can fall as well as increase rather quickly. A change in the average weight for height of a group suggests a change in energy balance.

There is no doubt that schoolchildren are now much bigger than they were early in this century. Periodic surveys by the London County Council showed, for example, that children aged 11 years were about 11 cm taller and 8−9 kg heavier in 1959 than they were in 1905. From 1959 to 1966, change was trivial, suggesting that the well-established secular trend towards tallness and heavinesss reached a maximum in 1954−9 (Cameron, 1979).

There is, however, strong evidence that differences in size at school age are largely determined by earlier growth patterns. Birthweight has a small but definite effect not only upon the size of schoolchildren but upon the size obtained in adult life (Miller *et al.,* 1972). After birth, growth is rather unstable up to about 1·5−2 years of age, after which it usually settles into a given "channel" of a standard growth chart. In an investigation in Newcastle (Fellowes *et al.,* 1979) about half the children changed "channels" during the first six months of life, falling to 0·4% in children aged 2 years or more. The changes in the early rate of growth were not associated with severity or duration of illnesses, and seem very likely to indicate the special importance of nutrition for growth during the first year or two after birth.

This is not unexpected since babies and young toddlers have little or no control over what they eat, and have to make a transition from a wholly liquid diet to an ordinary mixed diet, a process that involves many nutritional hazards. From about the age of 2 years until puberty, average growth curves of children are more or less parallel in large and small children, indicating that size has already been clearly differentiated by age 2 years; subsequent growth *rates* (increase per annum) are not greatly different. For this reason, I am inclined to doubt whether longitudinal studies of rate of growth in groups of children aged about 2−11 years are worthwhile, except in feeding experiments. Size attained probably gives most of the information we need from routine anthropometric surveys.

But age-specific averages derived from large heterogeneous populations do not tell the whole story. Children in different geographical areas and from different socio-economic backgrounds differ in size for age, at least in Britain. Those in the south of England tend to be bigger than those in the north. Rona and Altman (1977) found Scottish children in primary schools to be on average 2 cm shorter than English children. In both countries, children in the "upper" social classes were bigger, on average, than those from the "lower" classes (Rona *et al.,* 1978). In England, size of family (i.e. size of sibship) affected height in both the manual and non-manual groups. Such "social" factors, however, seemed to be less important than parental factors: tall parents tend to have tall children and vice versa. We do not, at present, know the extent to which the parental influence is genetic or due to the effects of the parental environment being continued into the next generation. Whatever the ultimate answers, the fact remains that the environmental hypothesis (which is strongly supported by the remarkable secular increase in growth of schoolchildren referred to above) spurs us to do something about unsatisfactory social conditions, whereas the genetic hypothesis may lead us into the rather sterile controversies of eugenics.

Having collected data on height and weight, we have to consider which form of analysis is likely to be most informative. In cross-sectional surveys, average values may fail to reveal important differences, because nutritional deterioration (for example) may be limited to relatively small groups of children in the most vulnerable groups, e.g. those from large families in the poorest social classes. Deterioration in such groups may bring about an increase in the proportion of very small children without significant change in overall mean values. We should therefore look at distributions as well as means and standard deviations. It is also worth noting that so-called "growth standards" ought to be used with great discretion in drawing conclusions of any kind. Such "standards" may be useful as yardsticks for purposes of comparison, but they do not necessarily imply target values which it is desirable to attain. It is particularly necessary to be wary of comparisons with standards which were derived from populations of different ethnic origin.

Finally, let us consider adults. A joint committe of the Department of Health and Social Security and Medical Research Council (1976) introduced its report by stating that: "We are unanimous in our belief that obesity is a hazard to health and a detriment to well-being". It believed that at least 20% of the population attempts to lose weight by one means or another, each year. Yet information on prevalence of obesity in Britain, and on whether it is tending to increase or decrease, is remarkably unsatisfactory. The committee commented on the lack of any nation-wide survey which would provide information about the overall prevalence of obesity and about regional, occupational or social class differences. It is good to know that the Department of Health and Social Security has commissioned a special study of heights and weights in adults, the result of which should provide a base-line with which future data can be compared.

Conclusions

It is not within my brief to discuss dietary surveys, but clearly nutritional surveillance is never complete without information on the quantity and quality of diets taken by the population. In Britain, we are fortunate that the National Food Survey has provided us with a continuous analysis of household food consumption during the past 40 years. Despite its limitations, I consider this to be a most valuable source of continuing information to the health services as well as to the food industry, and I hope that periodic attempts to eliminate it on the grounds of economy will continue to be resisted.

Dietary data based on consumption by individuals rather than by households, especially if accompanied by clinical and anthropometric data from the same individuals, would obviously be of even greater interest. But individual diet surveys are so difficult and expensive that I doubt if they can ever be undertaken routinely. *Ad hoc* surveys of special groups, such as children, should continue to be made when there is a good reason for doing so.

It may seem that I have advocated anthropometric measurements as the only satisfactory means of routine clinical evaluation of nutritional status; as stated, health statistics are of interest but of limited value and biochemical methods involve serious difficulties as regards ethics and interpretation. That remains my view with regard to *routine,* continuous monitoring. The institution of a national survey of growth and physique, in parallel with the National Food Survey, would be a considerable advance on what we have at present.

But, in addition, we will always need *ad hoc* studies when special problems arise. As society and its organization continue to change, we are bound to suspect that the nutrition of vulnerable groups is not what it should be. Examples from the past are the nutrition of old people, the feeding of infants and toddlers, and ill-health possibly due to malnutrition in some immigrant communities. Temporary surveillance procedures need to be instituted when such problems arise, the techniques being adapted to the nature of the problem. Controlled feeding experiments are of particular value. In such *ad hoc* research the specialized knowledge and facilities of university and research institutions should be utilized; and commissions should also be used to investigate and improve the methods of routine surveillance. On the whole, I think that routine surveillance is best undertaken directly by government departments. But only by regular interchange between scientific civil servants and independent research workers will points of view remain fresh and attitudes critical. The danger of any routine is that its thinking may become stale and its methodology outmoded. The Department of Health and Social Security in Britain has, fortunately for all of us, an excellent tradition of "outside consultation" in nutritional as in many other matters. But the government should consider that more might be done to extend the information it already assembles regularly through its own institutions, such as the National Food Survey, the General Household Survey, and the Office of Population Censuses and Surveys. My suggestion is a national survey of growth and physique.

References

Cameron, N. (1979) The growth of London schoolchildren 1904–1966: an analysis of secular trend and intra county variation. *Annals of Human Biology,* **6,** 505–25

Department of Health and Social Security (1973) "First Report by the Sub-Committee on Nutritional Surveillance". HMSO, London.

Department of Health and Social Security (1974) "Present-day Practice in Infant Feeding". Reports on Health and Social Subjects, No. 9. HMSO, London.

Department of Health and Social Security (1976) "Research on Obesity". HMSO, London.

Department of Health and Social Security (1980) "On the State of the Public Health. The Annual Report of the Chief Medical Officer of the Department of Health and Social Security for the year 1978". HMSO, London.

Department of Health and Social Security (1980) In preparation.

Fellowes, H. M., Hyttnen, C. A., Billewicz, W. Z. and Thomson, A. M. (1979) Health, growth and development of pre-school children in Newcastle upon Tyne. *Journal of Biosocial Science,* **11,** 411–24

Jelliffe, D. B. (1966) "The Assessment of the Nutritional Status of the Community." World Health Organization Monograph Series, No. 53. WHO, Geneva.

McKeown, T. and Record, R. G. (1962) Reasons for the decline of mortality in England and Wales during the nineteenth century. *Population Studies,* **16,** 94–122.

McLaren, D. S. (1974) The great protein fiasco. *Lancet,* **ii,** 93–6.

Miller, F. J. W., Billewicz, W. Z. and Thomson, A. M. (1972) Growth from birth to adult life of 422 Newcastle upon Tyne children. *British Journal of Preventative and Social Medicine,* **26,** 224–30.

Orr, J. B. (1937) "Food, Health and Income". Macmillan, London.

Rona, R. J. and Altman, D. G. (1977) National study of health and growth: standards of attained height, weight and triceps skinfold in English children 5 to 11 years old. *Annals of Human Biology,* **4,** 501–23.

Rona, R. J., Swan, A. V. and Altman, D. G. (1978) Social factors and height of primary school children in England and Scotland. *Journal of Epidemiology and Community Health,* **32,** 147–54.

The Potential Contribution of Commercial Market Research to Developing an Understanding of Food Habits and the Consumer

John McKenzie

Ilkley College, Ilkley, West Yorkshire

In a paper published in the British Nutrition Foundation's Nutrition Bulletin which aims to examine the nature and scope of social nutrition, I have made the point that we still lack any structured research activity to really aid our understanding of the causes of change in food habits, and the way in which we may initiate change in the interests of better nutrition (McKenzie, 1980).

In this same paper I have also suggested that whilst it is a necessary prerequisite to build up joint interest amongst scientists and social scientists and to provide appropriate opportunities for them to work together on social nutrition issues, what is crucially required is the development of a number of major integrated research programmes. Such programmes might individually cost of the order of £¼ million per year.

It would be silly to pretend that such budgets are likely to be generated within the foreseeable future. After all, the total income of the British Nutrition Foundation itself to cover all its activities in 1980 is just about £134,000.

But there is a very significant source of data which we should not discount. In 1979, £85 million was spent on commercial market research in the United Kingdom. Approximately £30 million was spent on behalf of the food, drink and tobacco industries, and a further significant sum went on studies related to the understanding of consumer purchasing behaviour in various fields (Simmons and Gordon, 1980) (Tables I and II).

This expenditure reflects the development of a dynamic research industry whose activities have grown significantly over the last ten years. Inevitably, we therefore need to ask whether the data available from these activities is likely to be of any relevance and whether it is possible to gain access to it for our purposes.

Preventive Nutrition and Society

Table I

Value of commissioned research in Great
Britain.

Year	£ million	Index of research turnover at current prices	Index of retail prices
1969	14–17	100	100
1973	31	200	136
1974	34	219	158
1975	36	232	196
1976	43	277	229
1977	55	355	257
1978	72	465	278
1979	85	549	330

Table II

Source of research revenue 1979.

Source	%
Food, drink and tobacco	35
Other manufacturing companies	15
Advertising agencies; media	15
Public sector	10
Service trades	5
Overseas	5
Miscellaneous	15

Does commercial market research really work?

It is often suggested that commerical market research does not match up to the rigour and quality of academic research and must, on these grounds, be discounted.

I do not find such arguments acceptable. I would suggest that such a view is primarily based upon claims made by scientists rather than social scientists, and reflects their "dis-ease" with social science techniques (even if used in an academic context) as with any fundamental criticisms of the viability of commercial market research.

Moreover, I believe it would be silly overall to suggest that the material derived from such an enormous commercial research expenditure could not, in some way, be utilized to aid our general understanding of patterns of food consumption and how these may be influenced in the interests of better health and nutrition. Indeed, it seems to me that most of the techniques related to issues such as product testing; consumer attitude; behaviour measurement; have achieved a depth and quality of technique as a result of commercial intervention which did not exist and could not have been developed from the relatively limited level of academic endeavours in these areas in the past.

To take the contrary view would be to suggest either that research which increases our understanding of brand and product fields has no wider relevance and cannot contribute in any way to general knowledge, or naively to imply that industry expends significant sums of money on meaningless, inadequate research that is not, in any sense, useful.

Thus, returning to our figure of £30 million plus, even if we discount work so significantly related to the detailed study of individual brands as to be valueless to us, duplicated work by competitors, and money going to the tobacco field, we are still left with perhaps £5 million of relevant and appropriate work being undertaken each year.

Some case studies

Commercial market research covers a wide range of activities. As far as our problems are concerned, useful data may be of three types:

    a) to aid understanding of particular markets;

    b) to identify consumer profiles and current behaviour patterns and suggest ways in which these may be influenced;

    c) to provide an understanding of a particular product field.

It may be helpful if I indicate by means of a case study involving two commercial studies, the sort of general data that may be obtained in this way. The study relates to the growth market of frozen foods and freezers.

Birds Eye (1980) have produced a detailed study of the market. They demonstrate that freezer ownership has grown from 19% in 1974 to nearly 43% in 1979. Of households in London 52% now own a freezer compared with 27% in Scotland. Predictably, size of freezer varies according to social class grouping (Fig. 1). Sales of fridge/freezers are now growing at the expense of solus freezers.

The market for frozen foods is also changing with a movement away from the traditional favourites of peas, fish fingers and beefburgers. But these products still lead the "top ten frozen food buys" (Table III).

Purchases are now tending to concentrate in the freezer department in the grocery store, whilst Birds Eye's proportion of the market is growing (Tables IV and V).

A recent IPC study set out to examine the relative influence of the husband/wife in inititating the purchase of major domestic durables and

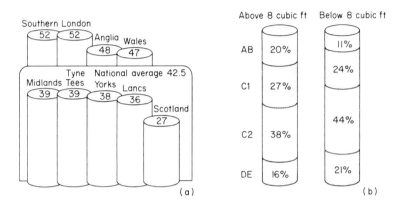

Figure 1   (a) Household freezer ownership by region at the end of 1979 (% home).
(b) Size of home freezers by social group. (Source: Birds Eye.)

Table III

The top ten frozen food buys: how products rank in percentage of total UK frozen foods spending (at consumer values). (Source: Birds Eye.)

	Freezer owners			Non-freezer owners	
	Product	% of spending		Product	% of spending
1.	Peas	11·4	1.	Fish fingers	11·5
2.	Beefburgers	10·8	2.	Peas	11·3
3.	Fish fingers	9·2	3.	Beefburgers	10·4
4.	Fish fillets	9·1	4.	Prepared meals (meat)	8·9
5.	Prepared meals (meat)	7·8	5.	Fish fillets	8·3
6.	Chips	6·2	6.	Crispy fish	5·8
7.	Meat pies	5·2	7.	Fish in sauce	4·8
8.	Other vegetables	4·6	8.	Breaded fish	4·3
9.	Meat pastries/savouries	3·9	9.	Meat pies	4·2
10.	Crispy fish	3·5	10.	Chips	3·6
	TOTAL	71·7		TOTAL	73·1

the key aspects they looked for (British Market Research Bureau, 1979). The survey demonstrated the significant role played by the housewife both in suggesting that the items should be purchased and in being present at the time of purchase (Table VI). The housewife is also likely both to refer to more product features than her spouse and indeed to give different ratings to them (Tables VII and VIII).

Table IV

Source of purchase of frozen foods by home freezer owners (expressed as a percentage of total expenditure on frozen foods).

	1977	1978	1979
Grocery freezer department	53	55	56
Specialist freezer centre	35	34	33
Other outlets	12	11	11

Table V

Birds Eye's share of the frozen food market, 1978/79.

	Total sales of Birds Eye	Sales through grocery outlets
1978	£ 233m (39%)	£ 202m (48%)
1979	£ 295m (41·5%)	£ 265 m (52%)

Table VI

Relative influence of wife/husband in the purchase of major domestic durables.

	Who first suggested item should be bought		Who was present when it was obtained		
	Wife	Husband	Wife only	Husband only	Both
	(%)	(%)	(%)	(%)	(%)
Vacuum cleaner	70	19	29	11	57
Spin dryer	64	26	28	17	55
Refrigerator	63	21	17	11	71
Washing machine	63	27	23	9	63
Cooker	59	27	22	5	72
Deep freeze	52	37	21	9	69

Table VII

Relative interest of husband/wife in product features

Average number of features mentioned	Cooker	Freezer	Fridge	Washing machine	Spin dryer	Vacuum cleaner
General features:						
by husband	5·6	6·0	5·8	5·5	5·4	4·6
by wife	6·3	6·2	6·1	6·3	6·3	5·1
Specific features:						
by husband	4·0	2·1	1·9	2·2	1·5	3·0
by wife	7·9	2·7	2·8	4·7	2·7	5·1

Table VIII

Comparison of relative importance of general features to husbands and wives.

	Vacuum cleaners	Refrigerators (inc. fridge-freezers)	Freezers	Washing machines	Cookers	Spin/tumble dryers
	(%)	(%)	(%)	(%)	(%)	(%)
Husbands						
Manufacturer's reputation	55	40	46	57	40	53
Price	68	74	80	67	66	64
Overall size	12	60	69	36	42	46
Appearance	10	29	12	14	37	18
Good servicing	40	46	50	56	41	47
Good guarantee	47	50	57	52	51	52
Safety	43	43	39	46	52	45
Reliability	66	64	70	64	53	59
Don't know/ not stated	10	7	6	13	8	13
Wives						
Manufacturer's reputation	55	41	49	63	48	57
Price	67	72	75	63	61	66
Overall size	21	68	75	43	52	60
Appearance	21	41	33	31	62	35
Good servicing	48	47	47	64	40	52
Good guarantee	50	52	56	58	50	55
Safety	42	41	42	53	58	52
Reliability	75	66	79	79	65	72
Don't know/ not stated	7	3	3	6	3	6

Evaluation

I have used these studies simply to provide examples of the way in which collection of data may help our understanding. But envisage such data collected and analysed in a much more comprehensive way and one may go at least some way to realizing the extent to which such data might help the growth of knowledge.

This is not, of course, to underestimate the political and technical difficulties likely to exist in obtaining the release of data from companies and making use of it.

Amongst the problems likely to emerge would be:

a) lack of comparability of data resulting from variance in research design implemented by different organizations;

b) difficulty in interpreting data collected with one objective in mind for a different set of objectives;

c) overcoming resistance to provision of data/suspicion of competitor use of it by industry.

However, much of the data is already available on a wider basis than is often realized. In summary, data is collected for three purposes:

a) to provide information to the public/media/specialist group; to sell a service; to support a product range; to sell a brand (such data is obviously *widely available* at least in summary form);

b) to provide information purchased on a syndicated basis for a particular group of companies/individuals (data usually available on a *limited access* basis especially for basic facts);

c) to isolate product or brand data for a particular company (material is mostly *confidential* unless "let out" in small amounts to aid brand sales but even then it is often out of context and, in consequence, difficult to interpret).

Even in the last-mentioned product/brand area the commercial significance of any data collected is usually lost over a two to three year time span and as such should enable the release of historical data.

Moreover, there are a number of past precedents in other areas to suggest such activities can get off the ground. Take for example the Marketing Communications Research Centre at the Cranfield School of Management. Here many firms are making available confidential material regarding their advertising and their evaluation in an attempt to understand the advertising process more fully and increase cost effectiveness.

Conclusions

Thus, I would recommend that the British Nutrition Foundation should very seriously consider trying to generate funds to set up a market research data bank. Given the support of the companies which comprise the membership of the Foundation, it ought to be possible to undertake a major screening activity of a wide range of data. At present, as well as being more realistic than trying to establish a research unit at a cost of say £¼ million per annum, it might be remarkably rewarding.

References

Birds Eye Business Report (1980).
British Market Research Bureau Survey Report for IPC (1979) In *Marketing,* September issue.
McKenzie, J. C. (1980) "What is Social Nutrition?" Nutrition Bulletin Vol. 5, Number 6. British Nutrition Foundation.
Simmons, M. and Gordon, L. (1980) Patterns of market research in the 1980s. In "Report of 23rd Annual Conference of Market Research Society".

The Unwilling Listener:
Some Lessons from an Advertising agency

Judith M. Lannon

J. Walter Thompson Company Limited, London

I would like to begin by quoting the March/April isssue of "Consumer Affairs" which dealt with the EEC symposium on Food, Food Technology and Nutrition Labelling held in London in March of 1980. The article, referring to John McKenzie's paper, said this:

> "Food habits are changing: for economic reasons, (improved capacity to buy the foods the individual wants), because society is constantly changing (parenthood, changing jobs or houses stimulate change), and because of the changing trends in food imagery." Professor McKenzie said he omitted nutrition education and advertising as factors, because of his primary thesis: "If food consumption patterns change, they usually change because the consumer wants them to. This is very different from persuasion to change because nutritionists, government agricultural economists or legislators want them to change".

and here I would add food manufacturers using mass media advertising.

There are two ways of interpreting these remarks. On the one hand, despair that nutritional education is a complete waste of time and should be abandoned altogether, and on the other, a recognition of the opportunities that a more realistic and focused view offers. After all, in democratic societies it is hardly surprising, and indeed a healthy state of affairs, for people to regard "persuaders"—whether in the form of nutritionists or advertisers—with some cynicism and suspicion.

I have titled this paper "The unwilling listener: some lessons from an advertising agency", because in much of the work we do, we have to deal with the fact either that people are not beating the manufacturers' doors down to purchase his product, or that a manufacturer is heavily in competition with B and C in order to increase his sales; and, as far as the customer is concerned, the products may be very similar. Consequently our skills are devoted to finding ways of conveying the advantages of our clients' products in ways that customers find interesting and persuasive enough to act on: to choose to pay for something that delivers enough of a reward for the customer to feel he has spent his money wisely.

In very similar ways, nutritionists are faced with how to deal with what can variously be described as apathy, conservatism, traditional resistance to change: there are many ways of explaining the fact that it is difficult to change food habits through education in the mass media. A small proportion of people will always actively seek out information; they will find it however obscurely it is hidden. But on a mass scale, the nutritionists' problems could be seen as similar to ours: how to communicate effectively to people who appear, on the face of it, at best moderately interested and at worst largely unwilling to listen.

The "popular" view of how advertising works or indeed any other form of persuasive communications through the mass media, is based on two models. One, I will call the "hammer and nail" theory: people will change their behaviour if enough information is hammered hard enough into people's heads—leading to an emphasis on facts and repetition. Or the "gratitude" theory: behaviour will be changed in response to entertainment provided by advertisement; or in the case of nutritionsts, people will change their behaviour in gratitude for learning the error of their ways.

Implicit in both these theories is the notion of advertising doing things *to* rather passive, dependent people. However, the issue is not what persuasive communications do *to* people, but rather what people do things *with* persuasive communications according to its perceived usefulness to them—because we are constantly faced with the question of why it is people learn some things and do not learn others.

In developing advertising we are looking for ways to present products that accord with people's own feelings, beliefs and needs: not with what we think they ought to know. Consequently, we have learned quite a lot about the ways people learn (or fail to) through mass media and how to increase the effectiveness of our communications as a result.

The need for a theory: how we believe persuasive communications work

Both of the "popular" models of communication I referred to earlier—the hammer and nail theory and the gratitude theory—are essentially *conversion* models and make certain assumptions about human behaviour. Firstly, the notion of a more or less rational decision making process; secondly, the consumer is seen as *seeking* information, assessing alternatives in a conscious and rational way; thirdly, that what the sender sends by way of a message is in fact received by the receiver: there is no discrepancy between the stimulus and the response. And finally there is the assumption of exaggerated power of either the media or the nature of the control.

None of these assumptions have much support either in common sense, academic literature or everyday working experience of advertisers. So what is the evidence? Behaviourists, cognitive theorists and mass communications theorists have contributed to a more realistic and useful notion of how persuasive communications work.

Reinforcement taken to mean reward is a fundamental concept in behavioural psychology and refers to the strengthening of a habit on the basis of reward. This is not a complete model since it ignores preconception, the subconscious and inter-personal influences. Nevertheless, it is obvious that advertising does function to "reward at a distance" by linking brands with desirable social roles. Thus imagery is important to recognize and food imagery in particular is something I will be returning to later.

Cognitive theorists stress resistance to change. Since attitudes do not exist in isolation, a complex situation results which exerts a consistent tendency to maintain balance and resist change. Many psychologists have produced evidence that individuals cannot tolerate too much inconsistency or imbalance between the effective and cognitive components and so will strive constantly to keep them in balance. An imbalance occurs when new information is received which then results either in a *rejection* of the information or a fragmentation so that inconsistent elements are isolated and compartmentalized so that the attitude exists intact.

What people do with food information often illustrates perfectly this phenomenon. The beliefs in conflict are, on the one hand, a sensual preference for the taste of the food, in conflict with information that says it is bad for me. Or the other way round: a dislike for the taste of something conflicting with information telling me it is good for me. In both cases the classic response, as predicted by psychological theory, is to ignore the incoming information as the imbalance is too great to accommodate by isolating it from the cognitive structure so that it is unable to affect action. The difficulties faced by road safety information, electricity conservation, alcoholic abuse information in changing behaviour on a mass scale, all offer examples where information coming from the mass media is in conflict with existing beliefs or habit pattern and it is far easier to reject or ignore the information than it is to change the habit.

Also of direct relevance is the work of *Gestalt psychologists* on perception. Their basic theory is that individuals do not attempt, even if it were physically possible, to perceive accurately every detail of the physical structure of objects viewed or to listen to every word of verbal communication. The mind takes the trouble to perceive *only as much as is necessary* to help classify the object or message; the rest is ignored as redundant. In other words things are perceived as wholes using minimum clues or symbols.

Mass communication theorists have made a further contribution. For many years much communication theory was based on there being an essentially *one way* flow of communications: the assumption that the public could be informed at will; that it is necessary only to put the "message" in front of them and it will be registered and indeed acted upon.

The enormous body of work produced by the mass communication theorists denies this. The consistent findings are that individuals selectively expose themselves to the media, selectively expose themselves to messages, selectively distort the content of messages, and selectively retain information. This is crucial to the understanding of ways to use mass media for educational purposes. Individuals are rarely information-*seeking* mechanisms but more often information-*scanning,* selecting the bits that fit and rejecting the rest.

So the most important picture of the process is to see consumers as active participants, without whose co-operation, educational communications can have no effect whatsoever. Therefore the traditional "transportation" model of sending and receiving messages as though they were a postal service should be replaced by a more accurate metaphor, "the resonance principle". The electronic metaphor is a familiar one: "strikes a chord", "rings a bell" are common phrases emphasizing *meaning* rather than merely registering the facts.

Implications for food communications

It may sound very depressing, if not tautological, that it is impossible to teach people things they do not already know or to induce actions they are not already committed to. I have overstated the point deliberately in order to shift preoccupations from the properties of the *stimulus*—in other words, from the content of what some people wish to communicate to other people—to where it properly belongs, the *people* who are being communicated to. What is in their minds already; why they should want to know this information; and how they might wish to use it. So that firstly we must thoroughly understand how people *choose* foods. And secondly, we must understand how people interpret communications about foods.

It may come as a surprise to hear from an advertising agency whose billings are mainly with food manufacturers, that very few campaigns have concentrated overtly on a nutritional platform. There are two main reasons

Table I

Priorities for different meal occasions. (Source: Findus Report: "Are they prepared?", 1975.)

	Midday meal with housewife alone	Meal for children after school	Meal with all the family	Meal with housewife and husband only
To be made from fresh, wholesome ingredients	4th	3rd	1st	2nd
Not to be a complicated recipe	1st	2nd =	2nd =	2nd =
To be inexpensive	1st	2nd	3rd	4th
To be quick and easy to prepare	1st	2nd	4th	3rd
To be well balanced for food value	4th	2nd =	1st	2nd =
To be fun/interesting to eat	3rd =	1st	3rd =	2nd
To be non-fattening	1st	4th	3rd	2nd
To be frozen	2nd =	2nd =	2nd =	1st

for this. The first is that women, by and large, do not choose brands of foods solely on the basis of their nutritional value. Many other criteria come into play according to the meal, e.g. speed, variety, price (Table I).

Secondly, and very much less obviously, the attitudes and beliefs that consumers bring to communications about nutrition are likely to distort information in quite unintended and often negative directions.

What, then, are some of the beliefs and attitudes people bring to communications about food?

General rules of nutrition rather than specific details, but here there is obviously a great deal of lip service paid to what one "ought to do" and what people say and do can be in contradiction. For example, women often speak of a concern for avoiding over-processed foods which is part of the general verbal approval of "natural" versus man-made food: that nothing is as good as natural and that refined products with no "synthetic" chemicals are "best". At the same time, frozen, packeted, tinned and dehydrated foods are regularly purchased because they satisfactorily fill other sorts of needs.

Knowledge and attitudes differ by age and social class. Older and less sophisticated people, when asked about nutrition, talk of basic food items—milk, eggs, cheese, meat, fish, greens—largely undifferentiated, but in unspecified ways "good for you". Not surprisingly, if they have not experienced dieting problems, their ears are likely to be closed as in the following remark: "There's no incentive...I'm quite happy...I've been eating like this, on and off for the past fifty years, so why change? I'm happy." Younger people, on the other hand, both as a function of relatively recent school exposure to nutritional information and also, in the case of women, as a result of slimming, have a more developed vocabulary and speak of both food components and food items. The following remark, inaccurate as it is, is typical: "Sugar doesn't fatten you, it is starch—your fats and your breads".

Although the evidence is generally that the level of awareness of the need for something defined as "a healthy diet" has increased considerably over the last ten years and that at least a proportion of the population has become actively interested, this higher awareness level alone does not necessarily lead to behaviour change. Indeed, it may be counter-productive. It is very common in our research to find support for what could be described as an anti-authority, wholesale rejection in order to avoid the inevitable conflicts in information coming from different sources: "First they say bread is good for you, then they say it's bad, butter used to be good now they say that is bad, I don't listen to any of them anymore."

Implicit in that remark are two problems facing education through the mass media: firstly, conflicting views means that no one knows and consequently "*I* know best about me". Secondly, a subtler theme: the resistance to being *hectored* and bullied by "them". The "them" is an emotional projection of authority: entirely unspecified as to a person or group of people but at a psychological level, a convenient excuse for rejecting the message.

Variety is widely valued. Women tend to assume that they are giving their families "goodness" if there is *variety* in the food they serve. Few believe that "one food contains everything" and so the day balances itself out if sufficient variety is provided. Why variety? The answer to this is complex and it is difficult to disentangle real reasons from rationalizations. What women tell us about the values of variety often tell us much more about the women than about the food. Firstly, many women, particularly working class women, are well aware of the comparative affluence they enjoy compared to that of their parents, and make remarks such as "I like to give them (children) a choice because I remember my childhood—we never had a choice—we had to eat what was put in front of us and every week it was the same: Monday sausages, Tuesday rissoles, etc., etc." Variety also gives women a sense that in some way they are relieving the boredom of catering: there may be a personal reward in trying new things although with children there are real limits to what is experimented with: more likely it is the choice of a "new Findus prepared meal" than an experiment from scratch.

Finally, and importantly, variety is a way of ensuring that the family gets a "balanced" meal from the nutritional standpoint. The following remark is typical: "It just comes across naturally. You go shopping and you have a certain amount of fruit and a certain amount of protein in the cheese and butter and meat and perhaps if you can afford it, a nice piece of fish. But it just comes naturally—you don't go out and say, well I must have that because it has got vitamin so-and-so in it."

Roles for advertising

The foregoing only touches on the state of mind and needs women bring to communications about food. But it helps provide a framework in which we can look at the kinds of roles that any specific communication about food can play. And I would suggest there are three basic roles as follows:

a) reminding people of what they have forgotten;
b) conveying new information/new uses;
c) food imagery: user, appropriate occasions; makers/source.

The reminder role

Advertising as a memory jogger—"don't forget the x, y, z"—is a very common role. However, that very simplistic concept overlooks a more subtle interpretation of the role, and that is to tap a more complex and deeply rooted set of beliefs and feelings, that have become submerged or superseded. A good example of a campaign designed to do this is a recent campaign for bread.

In the late seventies the Bread Marketing Group decided to commit money to advertising. The advertising task was to develop a campaign to help increase consumption of all bread; bread consumption had been steadily decreasing for many years. The first task was to establish why this was the case. Over-simplifying greatly, the reasons were several: competition from many other foods, particularly snack meals; price; but most surprisingly something that could almost be called *status*. Table II shows how women rate bread as a source of protein (low) and carbohydrates (high).

The advertising problem was to determine the most effective way of conveying facts about the food values of bread. The first problem the exploratory research addressed was: why is bread so undervalued and is there an underlying resistancce to accepting facts about the nutritional

Table II

Housewive's beliefs about food. The figures
given are percentages of the housewives
questioned who thought that a given
foodstuff was a souce of protein and/or
carbohydrate. (Source: Birds Eye/RBL, 1978.)

Source of Protein		Source of Carbohydrates	
Meat	49	Bread	48
Cheese	33	Potatoes	34
Eggs	29	Cakes	26
Fish	24	Sugar	18
Milk	16	Butter	15
Vegetables	7	Meat	14
Bread	5	Cheese	14

values of bread? The major findings were that most women claim to like, even "love" bread. At the same time they feel guilty about eating it because they believe it to contain only empty calories: bad values (fattening) or none at all rather than good values (protein source). But underlying all this were residual beliefs in bread's goodness, stemming from the meaning of the phrase "the staff of life", communal bread breaking rituals, and the role it played in their own childhood, symbolically linked with maternal warmth and security.

We experimented with a number of different ways of conveying what nutritionists told us about the food values of bread. Cold listings of food facts were either misinterpreted or misunderstood: strictly emotional appeals describing bread as "the staff of life" were perceived as evocative but insubstantial. The most convincing television presentation was a comparative claim using what women already knew about foods containing protein as a frame of reference: hence "penny for penny, bread is a cheaper source of protein than milk, eggs, cheese". As a piece of communication this comparison was the most meaningful way of increasing awareness of bread's protein value. It uses the context of bringing up a family which is reminiscent of their own childhood and the phrase "the family's greatest supporter" underlines the ubiquity of bread. It is the balance of emotional and factual information that makes the communication meaningful. Figures 1 and 2 are examples of two advertisements featured in Women's magazines.

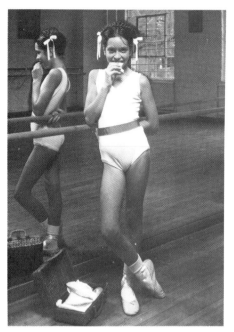

Figure 1

SHE THINKS HER SUPPORTERS ARE SMASHING.

Kids don't often like what's good for them. But there is one exception they never seem to say no to. Bread. They love it.

And it's just what they need when they're growing up.

Because bread nourishes and builds, supporting as it's always done.

Bread supports her with calcium for strong bones and teeth, and with essential iron and vitamin B1.

Bread supports her with energy — something children use lots of.

And, most importantly, bread supports her with body-building protein for growth.

So, for once, the thing she likes is the thing that's good for her.

Bread. It always has been. . . . It always will be. . . .

The family's greatest supporter.

THE FAMILY'S GREATEST SUPPORTER

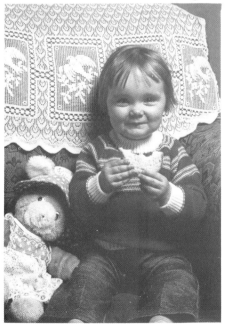

Figure 2

SHE NEEDS ALL THE SUPPORT SHE CAN GET.

Bread.

For every day of her young life.

Nourishing, building, supporting . . . as bread has always done.

Bread supports her with energy — and children use up lots of energy.

Bread supports her with calcium for strong bones, and with essential iron and vitamin B1.

And, most importantly, bread supports her with body-building protein for growth.

It's so easy to forget that a simple slice of bread contains all these ingredients, so vital for life.

Bread.

An everyday miracle that families have grown up on for thousands of years.

Bread is the family's greatest supporter.

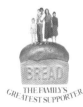

THE FAMILY'S GREATEST SUPPORTER

New information/new users

The research conducted in the bread case indicated that women actively wanted to believe bread was good and so were receptive to nutritional information in the right context: this is not always the case. More frequently communications fail because they tell people what the manufacturer finds most interesting: new ingredients; new methods; new research-based findings; new discoveries. They fail to distinguish between the manufacturer's pride in, say inventing a process for reducing dried soup preparation from 20 minutes to 5 minutes, or in making meat from soya beans, and what value this has to the consumer. The latter is currently a good example of spreading news of the manufacturer's triumph rather than translating this technological triumph into consumer terms. Soya products are on the market because they can be made, not because a *consumer's* need for them has been identified.

Often the problem is simpler and merely involves recognizing and using ordinary everyday consumer language rather than trying to impose manufacturer, technical, scientific or legal language. Cadburys and Rowntrees talk of count lines; chocolate lovers talk of chocolate bars. Nutritionists talk of fibre; ordinary people talk of roughage.

Consequently, a fundamental prerequisite to designing communications aimed at informing or spreading news is understanding and using what is in peoples' minds already, i.e. the *language* that already has meaning to an audience and therefore would be most readily understood.

A very much simpler form of new information caters to the interest in variety, recipes and creative cooking in general and has been widely employed in the advertising for eggs, milk and cheese. The nutritional values are well known and do not need spelling out. Consequently the role for advertising becomes one of giving useful recipe tips for these fundamental and potentially very versatile foods (Figs 3 and 4).

The role of food imagery

The word ''imagery'' may have negative associations to some, suggesting tricks employed by advertisers: dishonest illusion rather than honest fact. What I mean by food imagery, and what I would like to emphasize, are the elements beyond factual nutritional components that influence how food is chosen and used and how this imagery can be employed in food communications. This area requires the subtlest understanding of consumer psychology about what influences perceptions about food. There are at least three areas where new foods may find a foothold in existing attitudes and beliefs.

Crack a good breakfast

If you like an egg for breakfast, why not have two? Eggs don't cost much, and they make a great start to the day.

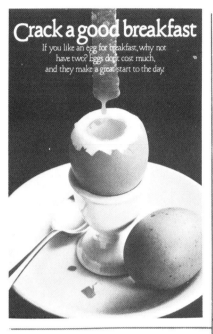

Crack a good lunch

Eggs Bayonnaise. For two. Fry 4oz bacon cut into thin strips, and ½lb of button mushrooms in butter. Stir in seasoning and 1 teaspoon of lemon juice. Separately fry 4 rounds of bread, top with fried eggs.
Arrange bacon and mushroom mixture around.

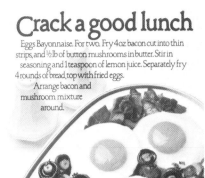

Crack a good supper

Oven Baked Omelette. For four. Heat oven to gas mark 6, 425°F. Butter a shallow oven-proof dish. Beat up six eggs and add grated cheese, sliced tomatoes, parsley and seasoning (or any tasty left-overs you prefer). Pour into dish and bake for 10 or 15 minutes till just set.

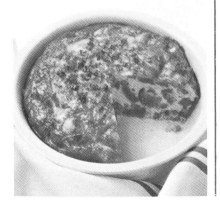

Crack a meal today

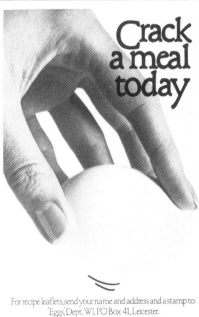

For recipe leaflets, send your name and address and a stamp to: 'Eggs', Dept. WI, PO Box 41, Leicester.

Figure 3

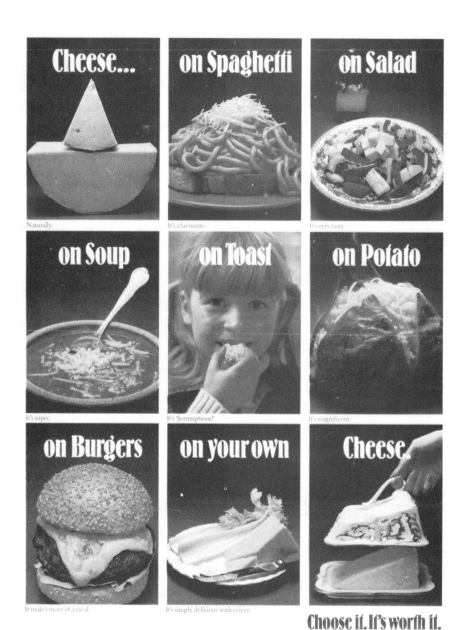

Figure 4b

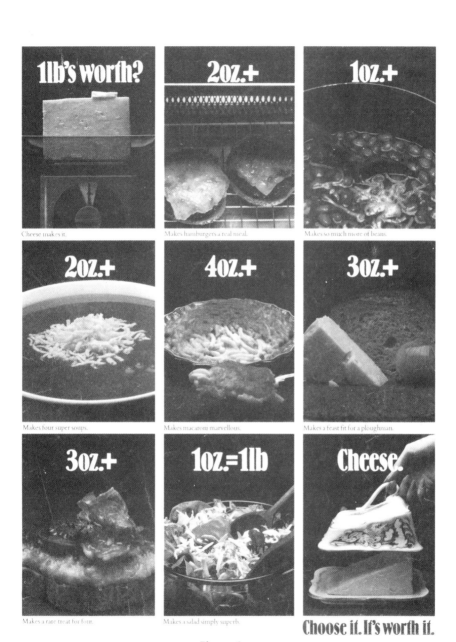

Figure 4a

Firstly, the link with traditional occasions and rituals. All societies have culturally and historically defined eating patterns: the ritual of Sunday lunch, breakfast patterns, night-time drinking, are obvious examples in this country. Brands such as Oxo link themselves firmly with traditional meat occasions and the importance of gravy, and brands like Horlicks have been closely tied with the psychological needs to punctuate the closing of the day with family consumption of hot bed-time drinks.

Secondly, the emotional needs that foods satisfy by symbolizing a wide range of added values: food as communication. Brands of chocolate such as After Eight and Black Magic satisfy much richer needs than merely a craving for sweets. Michael Nicod, in his paper "Gastronomically speaking: food studies as a medium of communication" (1980) and Stephen King's paper "Presentation and the choice of food" (1980) examine in considerable detail the crucial significance of the choice of food as symbols of very basic modes of communication between giver and receiver.

Thirdly, the importance of food *user* imagery and *source authority* in manufactured foods, and here I would like to quote more extended examples.

One of the major themes that our research amongst consumers shows is that people are suspicious of extremists and faddists and it is easy to imply this in communications unwittingly in an effort to emphasize food values. For instance, some years ago, anything remotely suggesting vegetarianism or health food evoked highly negative imagery. People interested in vegetarianism or who frequented health food shops were described as cranks, freaks, single spinsters, peculiar: in other words, not normal in the evaluative or statistical sense. Various developments have modified these perceptions although vegetarians are still regarded with some suspicion, especially male vegetarians—sexually impotent and ascetic. Consequently it is important that communications are designed so as not to imply that the *users* are faddish or freakish in any way.

Experience with Kellogg's All-Bran is characteristic of this kind of problem and advertising had been carefully designed and modified to appeal to a wide range of people. Originally the communications about the brand were highly factual, dominated by laxative claims (Fig. 5). The brand was used both by users of constipation remedies and people who feared constipation: a very small market indeed. By non-users, the brand was described as medicinal and clinical, and its users as peculiar or "odd", with an unhealthy pre-occupation with their insides: in a word, thoroughly abnormal ("not me") types of people. Figure 6 is an advertisement that communicated successfully with users aware of the functional virtues of cabbage, but non-users thought only of the taste of cabbage and the associations were almost wholly negative: school dinners, ugly smells,

CONSTIPATION SUFFERERS
should read this...

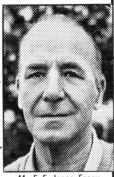

'I was recommended to try All-Bran... within two weeks I was back to normal...and have been regular ever since'

Mr. E. E. Jones, Essex

Mr. Jones took the advice of a friend and found that All-Bran relieved his old constipation problem.

There's no secret about All-Bran. It is an entirely natural and wholesome food which provides the roughage so often missing from modern diets . . . and so essential to keep your system regular. If you are constipated now, give All-Bran a ten-day trial. Or if you prefer something a little sweeter, try Kellogg's Bran Buds. They're just as effective. (If after ten days your condition still persists, you should consult your doctor.)

All-Bran or Bran Buds eaten regularly helps keep you free from constipation.

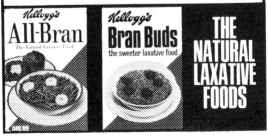

Figure 5

Will you be eating ¾lb. of cabbage today?

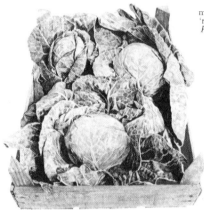

Not likely, is it? But that's how much you'd need, to match the amount of dietary fibre (the correct name for 'roughage') you get in just half a cereal bowlful (1½oz.) of *Kellogg's All-Bran* or *Kellogg's Bran Buds.*

The reason is simple. Wheat bran is an extremely rich source of dietary fibre.

Nowadays, experts say, many people are eating only a fraction of the dietary fibre people ate years ago. And recent research suggests that this 'low-fibre' diet is affecting not only our digestive system but our general health as well.

Happily, bran can fit easily into a family's everyday eating pattern. You can eat *Kellogg's All-Bran* or *Kellogg's Bran Buds* (the slightly sweeter version of *All-Bran*) at any time of day.

See the packets for enjoyable ideas – and for good ways of cooking and baking with them (soups, stews, cakes, all sorts of things).

You'll enjoy adding *Kellogg's* high-fibre wheat bran cereals to your menus.

Kellogg's **wheat bran cereals. For healthy eating.**

Figure 6

watery tasteless result. So that the message *received* was "cabbage is boring and so is All-Bran". The current advertising for All-Bran is aimed at a much wider audience and recognizes the need to emphasize general healthy living rather than drawing attention to a problem. Figures 7 and 8 are two examples of advertisements in this campaign.

Brown bread may be following a similar pattern. Brands of supermarket brown bread are coming onto the market and the aim of communications should be to make brown bread "normal" rather than to reinforce the moral virtues typically associated with it which tend to be translated into an unpleasant taste and rough (hairshirt) texture. Another example of food manufacturers *using* a trend, but, importantly, recognizing that people *know* brown bread is good for them, is what manufacturers must produce, and what communications must contain, is reassurance that the bread *tastes* good.

A third example is Flora magarine, a brand that recognized that women are concerned for their husband's health. Importantly, the advertising avoided concentrating on details of special ingredients and, more importantly for a brand wishing to gain widespread acceptance, avoided

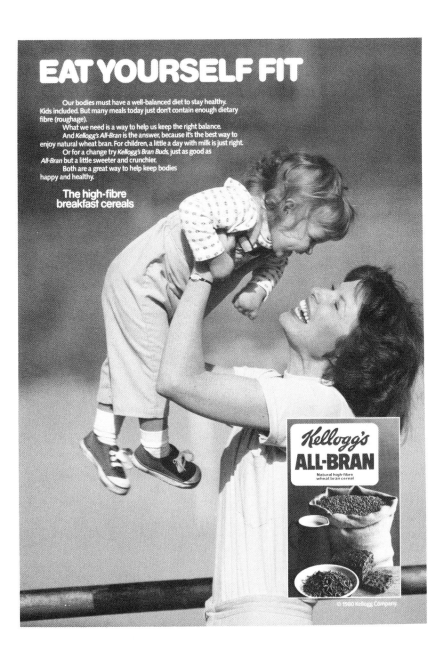

Figure 7

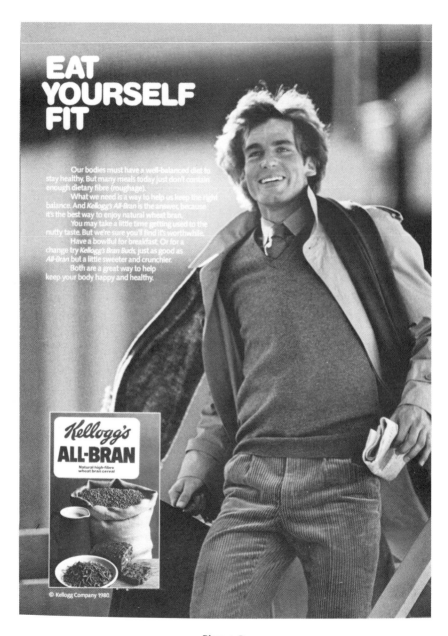

Figure 8

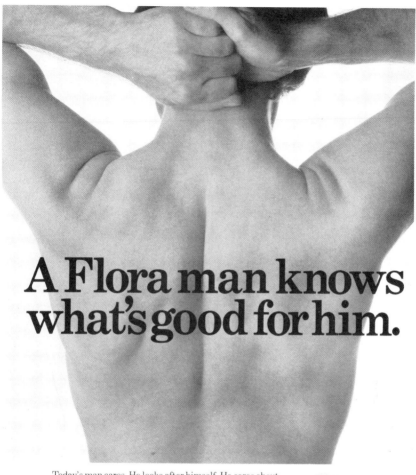

A Flora man knows what's good for him.

Today's man cares. He looks after himself. He cares about what he eats.

Flora is part of healthy eating. That's why you find more men becoming Flora men.

Their wives know they like that light, delicate taste.

And Flora is made with pure sunflower oil, so it's high in polyunsaturates.

Higher, in fact, than any other nationally available spread.

Is there a Flora man in your home?

Flora - high in polyunsaturates. The margarine for men.

Figure 9

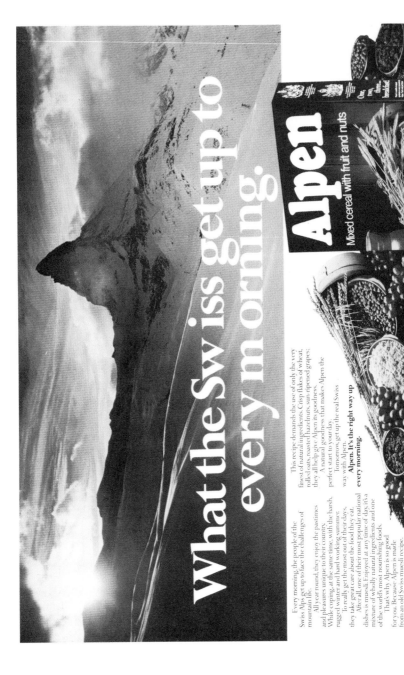

What the Swiss get up to every morning.

Every morning, the people of the Swiss Alps get up to face the challenges of mountain life.

All year round, they enjoy the pastimes and pleasures unique to their country. While coping, at the same time, with the harsh, rugged winter and hard working summer.

To really get the most out of their days, they take great care about the food they eat.

After all, one of their most popular national dishes is muesli. Enjoyed at any time of day, it's a mixture of wholly natural ingredients and one of the world's most nourishing foods.

That's why Alpen is so good for you. Because Alpen is made from an old Swiss muesli recipe.

This recipe demands the use of only the very finest of natural ingredients. Crisp flakes of wheat, rolled oats, roasted hazelnuts, sun-ripened grapes; they all help give Alpen its goodness.

A natural goodness that makes Alpen the perfect start to your day.

So tomorrow, get up the real Swiss way with Alpen.

Alpen. It's the right way up every morning.

Alpen
Mixed cereal with fruit and nuts

Figure 10

suggesting this was a brand for invalids, hypochondriacs or perhaps even more frightening, a preventive medicine; a brand to prevent heart attacks. The advertising takes great pains to stress the normal healthy life style that Flora suits rather than suggesting idiosyncratic morbidity (Fig. 9).

There is no doubt that an important trend in food purchasing is an interest in foreign foods and that a major role for advertising foods to a mass audience from other countries is to recognize the need for what could best be described as "safe exoticism" and to select appropriate imagery. This is often taken to mean that the foods themselves have to be reformulated in ways to make the flavours more bland, less sharp and distinctive because of a notion that English tastes are "conservative", which is often taken to mean bland. This may result in a serious misunderstanding of English tastes, which simple observation suggests are not bland at all: English mustard, Worcester sauce, the strong vinegar base in many condiments, sharp cheddars, strongly flavoured beers. What English consumers may respond to is not bland foods but rather conservative or more accurately *familiar* packaging and presentation. The successful introduction of Colman's packaged casserole mixes, Vesta meals, and Findus ranges illustrate the importance of presentation and packaging so as to present a balance between exoticism and familiarity: reassurance directed mainly at the understanding of the problems of women wishing to introduce unfamiliar foods to conservative husbands and children.

On the other hand, stereotypes of countries can be used overtly such as the reputation of the Swiss for concern with health used successfully by Ski yogurt and Alpen muesli-type cereal (Fig. 10).

Conclusions

Our experience is that communications about food work successfully and meaningfully, when they:

a) make connections with what people know already,
b) recognize the many and varied roles that foods play,
c) recognize the crucial importance of food imagery.

Food imagery covers the specific usage associations certain foods have, the sorts of people who use them (and the extent to which this effects their desirability), and the stereotypes held about various sources of authority.

References

Festinger, Leon (1957) "A Theory of Cognitive Dissonance." Harper and Row, New York.

Haskins, J. D. (1964) Factual recall as a measure of advertising effectiveness. *Journal of Advertising Research,* **4**, 1.

King, Stephen (1980) Presentation and the choice of food. *In* "Nutrition and Lifestyles", Proceedings of the First British Nutrition Foundation Annual Conference 1979, (Turner, M. R., ed.). Applied Science Publishers, London.

Koffka, K. (1935) "Principles of Gestalt Psychology". Harcourt, Brace and Company, New York.

Lowe, Martin (1980) Influence of changing lifestyles on food choice. *In* "Nutrition and Lifestyles", (Turner, M. R., ed.). Applied Science Publishers, London.

Nicod, Michael (1980) Gastronomically speaking: food studies as a medium of communication. *In* "Nutrition and Lifestyles", (Turner M. R. ed.) Applied Science Publishers, London.

Rosenberg, M. J. (1965) Inconsistency, arousal and reduction in attitude change. *In* "Current Studies in Social Psychology", (Steiner, I. D. and Fishbein, M., eds.) pp. 123–4. Holt, Rinehart and Winston, New York.

Rowan, John (1968) Selective perception and advertising research. Part 2. *ADMAP,* September.

Schwartz, Tony 61973) "The Responsive Chord". Anchor Press/Doubleday, Garden City, New York.

Lack of Response to Health Guidance among Heavy Drinkers

Douglas S. Leathar

University of Strathclyde, Glasgow

In Scotland, the national body responsible for health education, the Scottish Health Education Group (SHEG), makes extensive use of the mass media in educating the public on topics such as the responsible use of alcohol, the dangers of smoking, and the benefits to be obtained by adopting fitter, more positive life-styles. For the last two years or so, it has conducted a campaign which is designed to persuade people, particularly young manual workers, to monitor their regular consumption of alcohol. This takes the form of a 45 second television commercial, backed up by full page advertisements in the Scottish press. In research terms, the campaign represents the end product of a more systematic approach to the development of mass-media campaigns, jointly instigated by the SHEG and the Advertising Research Unit in the Department of Marketing at Strathclyde University. This paper describes the rationale behind this approach and, in tracing the history of the campaign development, discusses the practical and methodological problems encountered in directing advice to a sector of the population that is normally indifferent to any approach attempting to influence or comment on their life-styles.

A systematic approach to campaign development

Even though the image of advertising would sometimes suggest that striking campaigns are not difficult to create, the reality is somewhat different. In advertising, the clever idea is seldom simple, nor is it easily attained. Far from being the end-result of some solitary individual's brilliant invention, most major campaigns are the product of a great deal of concentrated effort, and of endless trial and error.

In this, research plays a crucial role. The key to successful campaign development probably lies in the extent to which "consumer" or audience feedback is taken into account in developing the material. Thus, from the moment the problem is identified, which in itself has usually involved considerable background research, the researcher and creative personnel in an agency are part of an integrated process continually discussing the material with its potential audience. It involves interviewing them in depth, often using specially developed projective techniques, at all stages of campaign development, from the earliest conceptual approaches right through to pre-testing and assessing the final end-product itself. As such, it is a continuous cyclical process, with the results of one stage amending and refining, and often radically changing, the next.

There are many reasons as to why such an approach has to be adopted. To begin with, communication is a very ambiguous process. Like beauty, it is very much in the eye of the beholder. Any single message, no matter how simple it may seem at face value, will almost invariably say different things to different people. Unfortunately from an advertiser's point of view, we see what our experience has taught us to see, which is not necessarily what is there in reality, nor what he wants or expects us to see.

Furthermore, it is often difficult to determine exactly what *is* seen. It is a curious paradox of advertising that what matters may not be what an advert ostensibly says; what may be more important is the impression it leaves behind. Most consumer advertising does not sell reality alone (if indeed it sells this at all); it also tries to project an attractive "image" which one wishes to associate with the product. This is a complex mixture of style, mood and "tone" which leaves behind an attractive or "warm" impression allowing people to identify with the main theme of the advertisement (Leathar and Davies, 1980).

For example, the success of certain brands of cigarette is possibly more strongly linked to the pleasant or exciting image one associates with them, than to the taste of the cigarette itself. Much beer advertising implicitly projects the warmth and sociability of in-pub drinking, reinforcing the excitement and manly image of Scottish drinking, rather than the intrinsic taste of the drink itself. Even apparently mundane products, such as washing powder, have carefully contrived images—the "mum who cares" in one famous brand is no advertising coincidence.

And finally, research is carried out to guard against any social class biases being reflected in the material. Though this is a problem with consumer advertising in general, it is nowhere more acute than in "official" advertising. This can bring with it an establishment air, which is often criticized for projecting a rather cold and distant middle class attitude, which is sometimes patronising and lacks empathy and understanding of the problems "real" people experience.

Clearly, all these issues require extensive researching among the appropriate audience for any particular campaign. Irrespective of how professional and experienced an advertiser may be, it is remarkably difficult to predict what is appropriate for any chosen audience and what is not. Campaigns are developed by professional people who often live and work in environments that are different from those of the audience for whom the material is designed. No matter how hard they may consciously try, they may find it difficult to empathize with values and life-styles different from their own; without research, their biases and pre-conceptions will almost certainly dominate the final material.

The development of the drinking self-monitoring material

The problem

It is the long-term aim of the SHEG to encourage a more responsible attitude towards the use of alcohol. In Scotland, the abuse of alcohol is a source of national concern. Estimates of its prevalence vary—according to the study and to the definition of what constitutes a problem—from the estimate of the Clayson Committee (Scottish Home and Health Department, 1973) that 2% of the adult population have a significant drinking problem, to a more recent estimate of around 10% (Saunders and Kershaw, 1978). Even by conservatively averaging these two estimates, this means that at least 450,000 adults in Scotland, out of a total population of about 5 million, seriously abuse alcohol (Scottish Council on Alcoholism, personal communication).

The effects of this abuse are considerable. Not only is the death rate of alcoholics twice as high as the general population (Scottish Health Education Unit,[1] 1976), but there are many other serious physical and social side-effects. Even twenty years ago, the suicide rate for alcoholics was 76 times that of the general population (Kessel and Grossman, 1961). In addition to liver cirrhosis, alcoholics are prone to stomach illnesses, vitamin deficiencies, and mental problems (SHEU,[1] 1976), In the social sphere, the serious abuse of alcohol is linked, for example, with marital difficulties, baby battering (SHEU, 1976) and children's behavioural difficulties (Nylander, 1960). In work terms, it is currently estimated to cost Scottish industry as a whole around £120 million in absenteeism, accidents and work quality. Convictions for drunkenness rose by 54% between 1958 and 1978 (Scottish Council on Alcoholism, in press) and admission to hospital for

[1]Now known as the Scottish Health Education Group.

alcoholism and alcoholic psychosis rose by 428% between 1956 and 1977 (Scottish Health Statistics, 1977).

All this is occurring within a rapidly rising consumption of alcohol world-wide (Kendall, 1979). In the UK, for example, annual per capita consumption of beer, spirits and wine rose 48, 149 and 296%, respectively, between 1955 and 1975 (McGuinness, 1979). Nor is the abuse of alcohol confined to the UK. World wide, there is considerable evidence that the proportion of any population with serious drinking problems is a logarithmic function of the average per capita consumption (Ledermann, 1956; de Lint, 1975). In other words, from the average consumption per head within a specific population, it is possible to predict the total number of those with serious drink problems. In the UK, even with its problems, consumption of alcohol is comparatively modest when analysed against international data: spirit and wine consumption per head of population is in the bottom quarter (Brewer's Society Handbook, 1978). In wine-growing countries, such as France, for example, it was estimated even 10 years ago that half the general hospital beds were occupied by people with alcohol-related illnesses (Brésard, 1969).

In Scotland, the most recent comprehensive study of the characteristics of drinkers (Dight, 1976) indicated that 74% of men and 46% of women drank at least once a week, and 88% of men and 68% of women regarded themselves as having reached the stage where drinking alcohol was a normal habit. Only 5% of men and 12% of women defined themselves as non-drinkers. Among men, there was a peak of drinking between 17 and 30 years of age, while for women it was between 31 and 50 years, and the evidence suggested that the younger the drinker the more likely he or she was to drink regularly. Furthermore, the survey highlighted that while the average amount drunk weekly by men and women was equivalent to 10 pints and 2½ pints of beer respectively, consumption was not normally distributed across the population. Instead, 30% of all alcohol drunk was consumed by only 3% of the population. All these were men, who tended to be aged 17−30 years; had manual occupations; whose fathers drank at least twice a week when they were young; and whose male friends were most likely to be heavy drinkers.

It is against this background that the SHEG has been promoting mass-media campaigns in the last few years. Previous publicity has focused primarily on the serious abuse of alcohol. Using press and TV advertising, it presented a series of "testimonials" from alcoholics, in which they described their life-style, their past history, and their eventual success in overcoming their problems. In addition to trying to make those with serious drinking problems aware of the dangers and encouraging them to seek advice, the campaign had the broader aim of educating the public about the signs and symptoms of potential alcoholism.

Following recent evidence that around 80% of the Scottish population are aware, at least to some extent, of the problems of alcoholism (Plant *et al.,* 1979), the SHEG is now focusing its attention on the long term process of the development of problem drinking. As alcohol is a drug of dependence, regular intake of sufficient quantities over the long term will result in a certain level of addiction, with consequent dependence. Though the exact quantities necessary to induce dependency are a matter of considerable academic dispute, and probably differ considerably from one individual to another, the view in Scotland is that, on average, a regular weekly intake of approximately 50 cl of absolute alcohol indicates a heavy drinker who is tending toward the long-term danger area. Anything over 70 cl weekly, which is equivalent to 35 pints of beer/lager or approximately 2½ bottles of whisky, indicates a level of drinking which probably has already resulted in serious problems (de Lint and Schmidt, 1971). The SHEG therefore wished to promote a campaign designed to educate the public, particularly young manual workers, to monitor their drinking levels, with the eventual aim of teaching them how to distinguish between responsible social drinking and more extensive drinking with more serious long-term consequences.

The method

Prior to briefing the advertising agency who were to handle this campaign, the SHEG designed the illustrated pilot press advertisement (Table I) This was done to explore the public's initial reaction to the concept of alcohol self-monitoring, and to offer developmental guidelines for the campaign.

The initial step was therefore to pre-test this pilot advertisement with a sample of its intended audience. In methodological terms, there are almost as many methods of doing this as there are imaginative minds to construct them. In general, however, they are all variants of two distinct types, technically known as "quantitative" and "qualitative" research. "Quantitative", as its name implies, involves interviewing a reasonable number of "consumers" (usually around one to two hundred), using a standard questionnaire with carefully worded questions asked in a prespecified order. "Qualitative" interviewing, on the other hand, is much less structured: it is really an in-depth free discussion, usually among groups of respondents who, at the direction of the group leader (a psychologist), discuss areas or topics rather than simply answering questions. It is thus possible to probe complex areas in considerable depth and use the inter-action among members to generate and develop original lines of enquiry.

In general, qualitative interviewing is probably the more suitable approach for this type of research. Unlike product advertising, much social

Table I

"Are you asking for it?"
(Text of a poster issued by the Scottish Health Education Unit.)

Before your next drink, we'd like to ask you a few questions—especially if you regularly drink 4 or 5 pints a day.

The answers may be important for you.

The fact is, we have trouble brewing in Scotland. It often starts with people who drink heavily, say 4−5 pints or 8 shorts most days. Those who normally have a fair amount of alcohol in their blood.

A surprising number—folk like yourself—become addicted without knowing it. Slowly but surely, they are becoming alcoholics.

So, we want you to think about your own drinking to find out whether you are a social drinker, or in the danger area.

Are you ready?

First you need to know how much alcohol you use. Fill in your score for last week, thinking really carefully about each day.

Here are the drinks values you'll need.

Drinks	Unit values
One glass of wine	1*
One tot spirits	1
One glass sherry/port	1
One pint lager/beer	2
One can special strength lager	3
One bottle wine	6
One bottle sherry	10
Half bottle spirits	15
One bottle spirits	30

*1 unit represents approx 1cl of absolute alcohol

Surprising when we are honest, how it mounts up.

If your total for the week is 50, or for any one day ten or more, you are without doubt a heavy drinker.

If you scored 70 plus, you're in the big league and alcohol has probably caused you some family or work problems already. You should accept our challenge to **stop** drinking completely for a fortnight to satisfy yourself that you can. But right now, you may want to find out more about what kind of drinker you are by ticking our seven yes/no boxes.

1 Do some of your friends drink more slowly than you? yes | no
2 Has anyone ever suggested you sometimes drink too much? yes | no
3 Are you drinking more, or stronger drinks than you used to? yes | no
4 Do you sometimes double your order for drinks at closing time? yes | no
5 Have you had a memory loss after a night's drinking? yes | no
6 At parties, do you often volunteer to serve the drinks? yes | no
7 Do you ever feel guilty about your drinking? yes | no

Even a couple of yes answers means your drinking is not as carefree or controlled as you might like to think.

More than two, especially with a high drinks score means that you must change things now, to limit the amount you drink.

If you are one of Scotland's big drinkers, you'll be a big spender too.

You'll be handing at least £10 a week, probably much more, over the counter to keep yourself and your friends happy, and your life and leisure are sure to be pint-shaped. So what can you do? How can you keep the respect of your friends when you are with them in everything but spirit?

What can you do?

If you drink heavily and have read this far, you're probably worried.

And we haven't even mentioned the health risks of excessive alcohol consumption, like liver cirrhosis, stomach trouble, nervous depression, and of course, the inevitable accidents.

If you have convinced yourself that you don't have alcoholic tendencies and don't need to stop drinking to find out for sure, then here are a few suggestions. They will limit your intake without cramping your style as the life and soul of the party.

1 Keep your eye on the clock—and make your drinks last. Don't get caught into buying rounds for people who are drinking faster than you.
2 Avoid beers with high alcohol content like special lager and if you drink spirits, dilute them with water or lemonade. Have something to eat while you are drinking.
3 Learn to say "No thanks" when you don't want a drink, and make it obvious that you mean what you say.
4 Spend some of the money you save on something else—a holiday weekend, clothes or some other goodies you have wanted for years.
5 Remember, there are alternatives to the pub—sports activities, cinema, hobbies or social clubs. You might even have a drink at home with your better half.

There is no doubt that alcohol can help you relax, and add to your enjoyment with friends. But if you go out night after night **just** to drink, something's wrong. Maybe it's more than just the taste that makes you do it.

Are **you** asking for it?

	Beer	Wine	Spirit	Cost to you
Sunday				
Monday				
Tuesday				
Wednesday				
Thursday				
Friday				
Saturday				

advertising is *negative*. It is often—especially in health education—"threatening" its audience. People are frequently being told to give up enjoyable activities such as smoking, for advantages which are long-term, possibly tenuous, and certainly not immediately enjoyable. Though benefits are being promoted, they are to be obtained by avoiding something which is itself attractive, instead of accomplishing something positive *in addition* to what is already done.

This means that such advertising can induce anxiety, and anxiety creates defensiveness (Leathar, 1980). In interviewing, therefore, one is continually operating in a world where genuine motivating factors and complex psychological rationalizations are often highly intertwined, sometimes apparently inextricably so. Penetrating these defences, and disentangling these factors one from the other, is a highly skilled interviewing task and the more global quantitative methods seldom provide the context for this to be successfully achieved.

For this research we interviewed 40 "heavy drinkers" (22 males, 18 females), defined as those who drank at least 25 pints of beer or the equivalent, on average, per week. All were in the 17–24 age group and of C2D socio-economic status. They were recruited by a professional market research interviewer and each was paid the standard £2 for participation. Each interview lasted approximately 1–1¼ hours and covered the determinants of drinking and its social context in addition to a discussion of the press advertisement itself. The interviews took place in Glasgow.

The pre-testing results

The advertisement's message

In many ways, this was a classic piece of pre-testing. It illustrated something which was objectively correct yet, in the eyes of the consumer, was saying the wrong things to the wrong people. The advertisement essentially encouraged the monitoring of absolute levels of alcohol drunk; from the discussions, however, it very clearly emerged that it is the context of drinking and associated attitudes towards it that should be monitored rather than the absolute levels themselves. In other words, to quote one respondent, "It is not how much you drink, but the *way* in which you drink it, *when* you drink it and *how* you drink it".

In the public's view, alcohol has either a primary or secondary function. In its primary role, it acts as a focus in its own right: a drug taken to change mood and relieve tension. In its secondary role, though it may have primary elements, it is part of other more social activities, not the sole focus of attention.

This means that the absolute amount drunk is not the only criterion one has to take into account. In the public's view, two people can drink the same amount weekly, but for entirely different reasons: alcohol consumption reflects a variety of attitudes towards it. Just because someone with serious drinking problems behaves in a particular way does not mean that those who *behave* in the same way have serious problems.

Thus by defining problem drinking by concentrating on the end-product, as this advertisement did, and ignoring the motivations behind it, one is regarding certain behaviour as invariably reflecting a certain problem. Instead positive answers to the behavioural-type questions defining problem drinking (column 2, questions 1–7) were seen to indicate a variety of situations and reasons for drinking, many of which reflected a fairly responsible attitude towards alcohol and were almost totally unrelated to problem drinking.

For example, question 1, "do some of your friends drink more slowly than you?" which is intended to capture the "between rounds" drinker, virtually demands a positive answer from all drinkers: "Everyone drinks at different rates so it is logical that some will drink more slowly". Question 3 "are you drinking more, or stronger, drinks than you used to?", intended to capture those who are becoming sensitized to alcohol and require more/stronger intake for the same psychological effect, covers virtually all younger drinkers who are physiologically maturing and consequently more able to tolerate alcohol. Similarly, most teenagers will spend more on alcohol than they did in previous years but this is simply a reflection of the fact that they are developing their careers and have a larger disposable income.

Most of the other questions were viewed in a similar light. Most males have experienced difficulties in remembering where they have been during a stag night (question 5); have occasionally drunk too much and have been told so (question 2); have almost invariably doubled the order for drinks at closing time since that is an intrinsic part of the system of round-buying and almost a fact of life (question 4); and have inevitably felt guilty the morning after the night before (question 7).

As a result almost everyone, social and problem drinkers alike, would answer "yes" to the majority of the questions. They were not in themselves felt to indicate problem drinking, but have to be interpreted within the context of how one drinks, one's attitude towards drinking and its role in one's own life-style.

To the respondents, the key life-style indicators of problem drinking encompassed two broad areas.

1) *Daily versus weekend drinking:* Most respondents confined their drinking to the end of the week, from Thursday to Sunday. Drinking earlier in the week could easily take place, but for fairly obvious reasons—celebrations, special occasions, or just for "a change from the usual staying at home and watching the telly". With weekend drinking, and with the pub as the social focal point, most people could easily reach the "danger" level of 25 pints of beer. Yet the same total could be reached by those who drank a much lower amount each evening, but did so consistently throughout the week. *They* were felt to be the potential problem group, especially if they went to the pub virtually all the time just to drink. They often did so alone or, if with others, engaged in minimal social conversation. As one perceptive respondent noted:

> If you go into pubs like the H—, you can see guys come out of their work, walk in and they're not talking to anyone. They just stand at the bar, have 3 pints and then go home, get changed, come back and get started. If you really tested these guys you would be hard pushed to get them up to 30 pints, but I would consider them twice the drinker I am. We all go out with people, enjoying themselves, but they're not.

Consequently, this feeling that it was the attitude behind the drinking rather than the absolute amount drunk made a mockery of the advertisement's perceived claim that someone was a heavy problem drinker "if he had a score for 1 day of 10 or more": one could, in the public's view, have a "healthy" attitude towards drink consuming double this amount on a Friday night and an unhealthy attitude drinking less than this if it represented committed regular nightly drinking.

2) *Regularity of drinking:* "Normal" (and hence less at risk) social drinkers were seen to be those who fitted drinking in the pub to their life-style, not vice versa. Thus if circumstances changed and other factors became more important, they had the ability to adjust not only when they drank but how much they drank. Busy periods or overtime at work; studying for examinations; lack of money; even simply feeling like not drinking; all influenced the extent to which one regularly drank. Thus "normal" regular social drinking is, in a sense, irregular: it varies according to personal circumstances. The more serious, more at risk drinker, on the other hand, was seen to be more accustomed to adjusting his life-style to accommodate his priority of drinking on a regular basis.

Both these points illustrate, essentially, that the socially "safe" drinker is felt to be one who can maintain his priorities. He adjusts his drinking to fit into these priorities: those who are more at risk are more inclined to change their priorities to accommodate drinking. Consequently "maintaining priorities within one's own life-style" was the key concept to monitor in the drinking area, not just frequency. The emphasis, therefore, was not a static one, but on monitoring life-style changes over time.

Though these priorities are obviously different for each individual, commonly stated examples for the average person were:

a) Not missing work on a regular basis, though on certain socially sanctioned occasions this was acceptable, e.g. at Hogmanay, after a stag party.

b) Maintaining a regular consistent standard of work.

c) Not drinking to the exclusion of eating. At lunchtime the more serious drinker would drink without having anything to eat.

d) Not missing meals in order to go drinking, e.g. in the evening.

e) Not incurring financial strain when drinking. Reducing drinking levels or not going to the pub at a time of financial hardship.

f) Not drinking on a regular basis outside the round, though exceptions are permitted, e.g. being particularly thirsty during hot weather.

g) Not losing the respect of "your mates" through "your drinking going over the score."

Thus the general conclusion to be drawn from respondents' comments was that they felt that the advertisement concentrated on the wrong aspect of drinking and dealt with the consequences not the determinants of drinking. As one respondent observed, "It is like assuming that all football supporters are hooligans simply because they go to football matches."

By concentrating on absolute levels drunk and basically ignoring attitudinal and motivational factors, the advertisement focused its attention on those who drank fairly heavily but who regarded themselves, probably justifiably, as having a fairly responsible attitude towards drink. In other words, it made the classic communication error of directing a "correct" message towards the wrong target group.

The advertisement's tone and image

As was stated earlier, part of the function of pre-testing is to examine the less obvious effects of tone, image, style, etc. in addition to what the advertisement overtly says.

In general, people have difficulty in verbalizing about abstract concepts such as images. One way of overcoming this problem is to try to get respondents to relate to a concrete representation of the image. For example, one can ask them to imagine that the poster is a person and get them to describe the type of person they think it is. Such "projective" questions, though on the surface unusual and totally unrelated to the topic being discussed, can, in fact, offer insight into consumer perceptions that more direct questions cannot provide.

This advertisement, as a person, was feminine (an interesting comment in view of the masculine image of drinking), rather cold, grey and impersonal, yet possibly with a hidden sense of humour. She was slightly moralistic and reproving, having much in common with the traditional image of the elderly spinster schoolteacher. Given time and effort one could probably get to like her and underneath her cold exterior lay to some extent a sense of compassion and sympathy. She was not, however, "your kind-hearted mother or granny".

Some of these images undoubtedly derived from the type of advertisement this had to be. By presenting a fairly complex argument, the proportion of copy to visual presentation was many times greater than for most other advertisements. Under certain circumstances, a copy advertisement *can* be appealing, if it is of high relevance or, as for example with the SHEG's recent alcoholism testimonials, tells a particularly interesting story. But usually too many words detract from the appeal, particularly if it lacks impact by projecting a threatening message in the first place.

Then there is the language itself. Generally, to communicate successfully, one has to communicate in the style of the audience, or in absolutely neutral language; this advertisement, in many respects, fell seriously short of what was required. Phrases such as "have a drink at home with your better half", "have alcoholic tendencies", "some other goodies", "your life and leisure are pint shaped", all jarred. Concepts such as "volunteering to serve the drinks at parties", "caught into buying rounds", "spend some of the money on something else," "there are other alternatives to the pub", did not reflect the life-style and social norms of the typical young Glaswegian. Similarly, the humour, with its clever play upon words, such as "leisure is pint shaped", "with them in everything but spirit", "trouble brewing in Scotland", failed to imitate the Glaswegian sense of humour, which is basically depends for its effect on the perceptive observations of others. In fact, the "trouble brewing in Scotland" line disorientated those who interpreted it literally, leading to their seeing the "are you asking for it" heading as a plea by the brewers for understanding and sympathy for possible beer/lager shortages in hot weather!

All these aspects, each individually trivial little details, combined to create an overwhelmingly unattractive effect. Though objectively none of the information was incorrect, it failed to communicate with its potential audience, simply because it lacked empathy and understanding of their life-style.

The final campaign

The pre-testing therefore provided a great deal of useful information on both the concept of alcohol self-monitoring and how to communicate it to the public. In particular, it highlighted certain features which had to be heavily emphasized in the final campaign.

a) The message had to be directed towards heavy drinkers *who were changing (or had already changed) their priorities as a result of their drinking*. Thus frequency of drinking was presented within a context *not* in isolation.

b) The theme had to be believable, demonstrating behaviour going beyond the accepted "norms" of the typical, responsible social drinker. Such abnormal behaviour had to be defined by the person's own reference group or friends, not through standards externally imposed by some anonymous authority. Equally, the theme had to show behaviour which indicated the beginnings of the slide towards problem drinking, not behaviour at the confirmed alcoholic, "point-of-no-return", stage.

c) The context presented had to relate to the audience's own life-style. It had to understand and identify with them, and talk about "real" social situations to which they could relate.

d) In common with SHEG campaigns, it had to present a message which was serious, but not threatening to the point of inducing defensiveness. As such, it had to attract and maintain attention, while promoting an unattractive but relevant message.

e) The message, and in particular the language, had to be free from any middle class or official "tone".

The 45 second television commercial which formed the basis of the campaign presented a real life, in-pub scenario. It showed a crowd of football supporters in a typical pub prior to an important, all-ticket match. The action focused on a small good-natured group who clearly were drinking but not to excess, simply having the "normal couple of pints before a big match". One of the group was obviously in a far worse physical state than the others, indicating that he had been drinking much more extensively. As the time came for the group to leave the pub for the match, he attempted, against their wishes, to buy another round. After discovering that he had run out of money, he initially tried to buy the drink "on the slate", but was refused. He was then approached by a seedy-looking character who had watched the action, and offered "a fiver for your ticket". At this point, his friends rallied round, trying to reason with him, but in spite of this the ticket was sold. The action closed with the central character alone in the pub with his money but no ticket and no friends—and also no drink, since, in a symbolic gesture the pub closed before he could spend the money.

In conceptual terms, the message contained several important features. The main character started as a normal, ordinary person, one of a typical "group of mates". Thus initially he was not rejected, nor did he conform to the obvious stereotype of a potential alcoholic. He then rapidly showed the effects of alcohol, indicating that its consumption was outside the limits of normal accepted behaviour, a process reinforced by his general attitude and by his determination to carry on drinking. His attempt to buy drink on credit; his selling the ticket which previously was highly valued; and the statement by one of his friends that he would miss the match *again* (thereby implying that this was not an isolated, perhaps forgivable, incident) indicated both the abnormal priority given to drinking and the *changing* of priorities to facilitate it.

Ultimately, he stood outside the group, in physical and symbolic isolation, indicating not only that he rejected *their* standards, but that they rejected *his*. The implication, however, was that the rejection might only have been temporary, and the group might attempt, as it had done in the past, to bring his behaviour back to within their standards. He was therefore presented as someone at the edge of their circle, vacillating between acceptance and rejection. All this was reinforced by the punchline —"If drink has become the most important thing in your life, think again" —which emphasized the potential alcoholic's change in priorities.

In terms of the creative presentation of the message, too, the style used was a complete departure from that previously pre-tested. The context was clearly a normal life-style, and the characters were ordinary, young "working class" football supporters who might be found in any pub prior to a big match. The language was carefully scripted to be "typical consumer", with a strong Glaswegian bias, and all references to official language, attitude and tone were systematically removed.

The commercial has been periodically transmitted throughout the last two years, and backed up by the illustrated newspaper advertisement (Fig. 1). As this was intended to complement the television campaign, it had some elements in common (for example, the final punchline) and others which were extensions of the commercial's basic theme. Being in a different advertising medium, the conceptual approach was different. Often, the advantages of more extensive argument in a press advertisement are outweighed by the difficulties of attracting attention and presenting an appealing image: the television commercial has a more captive audience than is possible in press advertising, which has a greater element of selective perception.

The first problem was therefore to attract and then maintain attention. Attracting attention is usually a function of the main headline, visual presentation and general image created. As this advertisement was essentially a verbal one, its appeal had to be a function of the photograph illustrated, and in particular, of the headline. To emphasize the connection between the advertisement and the television campaign, the picture featured the television commercial's central character drinking in a pub. To

Can you hold your bevvy or is your bevvy holding you?

O.K. you drink. So do most people. But the Scots drink more than most people.
And that puts us in Europe's premier league for drinking problems.
    Great. So we're amongst the leaders in something—kind of makes up for the World Cup doesn't it?
    Come on. Who's kidding who? Just answer honestly the quiz below then check your rating at the end. You'll probably have a great laugh when you all do it in the pub. But who will the laugh really be on if you don't like the results.

1. Have you ever been refused a drink because the barman reckoned you'd had enough?
                                         YES NO
2. Do you miss the disco or the match because you get too drunk too early?   YES NO
3. When you were hard-up, have you ever borrowed money to go drinking or gone out broke hoping that someone would stand his hand?   YES NO
4. Apart from a special celebration like a stag night—do you get the shakes the morning after a bevvy?   YES NO
5. Are you running into trouble at work because of the night before?   YES NO
6. Do the mates keep nagging you that your drinking is over the score?   YES NO
7. Has drink ever got you into bother with the police or your family?   YES NO

Every yes you collected is just a warning. The more yes's you got, the greater your chance of having a drink problem. There's no magic number of yes's or no's which says you're O.K. or you're not O.K. It's up to you to know the score.

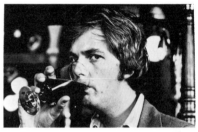

The Pub Test—For people who are drinking while reading this. If you think none of these situations applies to you, try believing your own eyes. Below are 16 squares, 6 have letters in them, the rest have the numbers 1 to 10. Disregard the letters and working from 1 to 10 touch each numbered square one after the other. Time Yourself.

10	7	B	3
A	9	C	1
4	F	6	D
E	8	2	5

    If you took 10 seconds, Congratulations. Sober it can be done in 7 seconds.
    If you took more than 10 seconds, you've got problems.
    Now. Who's holding who?

If drink has become the most important thing in your life – think again.

ŤŤ Scottish Health Education Unit, Dept. DS 1, Freepost, Edinburgh EH12 0PQ. (No stamp required)

Figure 1

overcome criticisms that the language in the initial advertisement was official and middle class, the headline was completely reconstructed, and written in colloquial Glaswegian which had a much greater impact (for English readers, "bevvy" is Glaswegian for drink!).

To maintain attention, the advertisement contained a quiz which was designed to create interest and add some lightness to a serious message which might otherwise have become too threatening. Based on American research, it invited the reader to measure his reaction time when under the influence of alcohol. Thus it not only acted as an interesting aspect in its own right, it had the subsidiary effect of illustrating the rather insidious effect of alcohol, since few of those interviewed believed that they were incapable of completing it in the stated time when under the influence of drink.

In between the headline and this quiz was contained the "serious" part of the advertisement. As in the previous version, this took the form of inviting "YES/NO" answers to several questions. Unlike the previous set, however, they were constructed to be such that normal social drinkers would be unlikely to respond to them, even if they drank fairly heavily. Thus they made exceptions for occasional lapses—such as getting blindly drunk during a stag party—and concentrated on examples of regular excessive drinking. Behaviour such as borrowing money for drinking, and regular occurrences of going beyond accepted standards, such as getting drunk too early at a disco or being nagged by one's mates, were featured, as were some of the potentially serious consequences, such as getting the "shakes" or being in trouble with the police or one's family. Finally, unlike the previous advertisement, no safe standards were implied. Instead, it appealed to the person's own judgement, since the pre-testing indicated that people with potential problems were perfectly capable of recognizing their behaviour *if* it were correctly presented to them.

Conclusion

The campaign as a whole, therefore, tried to emphasize examples of the gradually changing priorities the problem drinker adopts over the long term. As such, it featured how he starts within the accepted norms of his friends, and slowly moves outside them. It did make the assumption, however, that these standards reflect socially responsible drinking, and that people can recognize behaviour which deviates from them.

All through this research, it was a feature of the interviewing that people are more capable of recognizing behaviour which deviates from the norm than they sometimes are given credit for. Nevertheless, it may be that their standards contain a misguided belief about "safe" levels, even though other priority criteria are being met.

Future health education will undoubtedly develop this area, as it is only through the long-term creation of self-imposed norms that socially responsible drinking can ever be achieved. In order to do this, however, one has to establish a baseline context in which people are educated about the need to maintain priorities within the life-style they adopt. This would seem a more immediate objective; otherwise, as the original pre-testing only too clearly demonstrated, there is a risk of promoting a "correct" message within an incompatible, non-receptive context.

References

Brésard, M. (1969) *Revue d'Alcoolisme,* **15,** 81.

The Brewers Society Statistical Handbook (1978) Brewing Publications, London.

de Lint, J. and Schmidt, W. (1971) Consumption averages and alcoholism prevalences: a brief review of epidemiological investigations, *British Journal of Addiction,* **66,** 97–107.

de Lint, J. (1975) Current trends in the prevalence of excessive alcohol use and alcohol-related health damage. *British Journal of Addiction*, **70,** 3–13.

Dight, S. E. (1976) "Scottish Drinking Habits". A survey carried out for the Scottish Home and Health Department, Office of Population Censuses and Surveys. HMSO, London.

Kendall, R. E. (1979) Alcoholism: a medical or a political problem. *British Medical Journal,* **1,** 367–71.

Kessel, N. and Grossman, G. (1961) Suicide in alcoholics. *British Medical Journal,* **2,** 1671–2.

Leathar, D. S. and Davies, J. K. (1980) The role of images in health communication. *In* "Marketing into the 80s", Proceedings of the Joint EAARM/MEG Conference, Edinburgh, pp. 410–17.

Leathar, D. S. (1980) Defence-inducing advertising. *In* Proceedings of the 33rd ESOMAR Congress, Monte-Carlo, pp. 153–73.

Ledermann, S. (1956) "Alcool, Alcoolisme, Alcoolisation", Institut National d'Etudes Demographiques, Travaux et Documents, Cahier no. 29. Presses Universitaires de France, Paris.

McGuinness, A. (1979) "An Econometric Analysis of Total Demand for Alcoholic Beverages in the UK, 1955–75". Scottish Health Education Unit, Edinburgh.

Nylander, I. (1960) Children of alcoholic fathers. *Acta Paediatrica Scandinavica,* **49,** Supplement 121.

Plant, M. A., Pirie, Fiona and Kreitman, N. (1979) Evaluation of the Scottish Health Education Unit's 1976 Campaign on Alcoholism. *Social Psychiatry,* **14,** 11–24.

Saunders, W. M. and Kershaw, P. W. (1978) The prevalence of problem drinking and alcoholism in the West of Scotland. *British Journal of Psychiatry,* **133,** 493–9.

Scottish Council on Alcoholism (1981) "Employment and Drink". Edinburgh.
Scottish Health Education Unit (1976) "Understanding Alcohol and Alcoholism". Edinburgh.
"Scottish Health Statistics" (1977) HMSO, London.
Scottish Home and Health Department (1973) "Report of the Departmental Committee on Scottish Licensing Law" (The Clayson Report). HMSO, London.

The Role of Health Professionals in Nutrition Education

Sylvia Robert-Sargeant

British Nutrition Foundation, London

It has been said that education and politics cannot be separate because any educational innovator has also to be a skilled negotiator. One must also understand that education will often reflect what others desire from the system.

In this context, one must consider the changes that have taken place in our society in relation to health. The patterns of disease are changing with more chronic illness, disabled people surviving longer, mental illness on the increase, and more malignant diseases. The consumers themselves are also changing; their expectations are greater, they are better informed and their

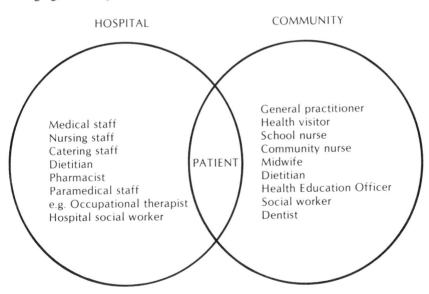

HOSPITAL   COMMUNITY

Medical staff
Nursing staff
Catering staff
Dietitian
Pharmacist
Paramedical staff
e.g. Occupational therapist
Hospital social worker

PATIENT

General practitioner
Health visitor
School nurse
Community nurse
Midwife
Dietitian
Health Education Officer
Social worker
Dentist

Figure 1   Health-care professionals

standard of living has improved. It is essential, therefore, when monitoring and developing health-care systems that these messages are effectively translated to ensure that the consumer's needs are taken into account. Health care cannot be given in isolation; it must respond to the pressures and needs of society. Failure to do so will inevitably result in problems. As I have said already, patterns of disease are changing; most modern diseases have a multifactorial aetiology often with bad nutrition as one factor. Evolution in the content of the training courses must reflect these changes in the pattern of disease if health-care professionals are to be able to operate effectively.

In this chapter I shall be looking at the actual and potential role of those health-care professionals most involved with giving nutritional advice to the consumer (Fig. 1).

Doctors

Despite evolution within other health-care professions, doctors, particularly general practitioners, remain the most available, and are the first point of access to a health-care system. They are the modern equivalent of religious leaders of bygone days but instead of a flock they have their list of patients.

When some medical students were asked recently how nutrition was covered in their training the reply was, after a pause, "fag ends".

When they explained one could understand this comment (Fig. 2; WHO, 1974). From the figure it can be seen that nutrition may be taught in the pre-clinical course by anyone from a biochemist to a clinical pathologist. In the clinical part of the syllabus virtually no medical school offers separate instruction in nutrition or dietetics.

A recent survey carried out by Fieldhouse (1979) showed in more detail where GPs had received their knowledge of nutrition:

Pre-clinically: separate nutrition course	5%
Pre-clinically: part of other course	34%
During clinical training	29%
Post registration	5%

Surely we must see in the future that nutrition and dietetics are an integral component of the medical curriculum, and ensure that it is presented to the medical student in such a manner that he or she can make use of that knowledge in medical practice.

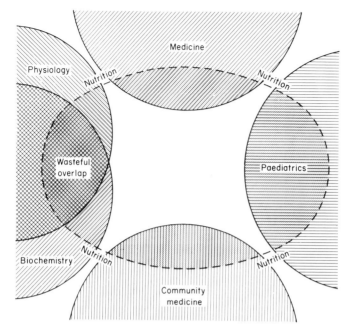

Figure 2 The relationship of nutrition to existing departments in a medical school.

Even within the framework of post-graduate education the provision of sessions on nutrition has been very piecemeal (Rhodes, 1980).

The recommendations of the International Union of Nutritional Sciences' Committee on Nutrition Education in Medical Faculties, as cited by the British Nutrition Foundation, Department of Health and Social Security and Health Education Council in their joint report, Nutrition Education (1977) stated that "active efforts are needed to support post-graduate education which would keep the practising physician informed of advances in nutrition knowledge."

Let us hope that the development of schools of graduate medicine (which are a logical step forward from the under-graduate schools), will allow nutrition and its application to be included as an essential part of graduate training.

I emphasize *essential* because the potential benefits of reducing the prevalence of disease are enormous in both personal and financial terms and, as was stated earlier, the GP is the obvious person to initiate preventive action.

Let us look at one example that has already been quoted—the cost of constipation to the National Health Service—which was about £20 million in 1979 (Laing, this volume). The principles of a high fibre diet are not too difficult for any GP to explain but in most cases a prescription for laxatives seems to be the quicker and easier solution.

Caterers

Nutrition may not exactly be a dirty word amongst caterers, but it is well down the list of priorities for the vast majority. Many will go so far as to say that their job is simply to meet the demand of the customer and to do so at a profit.

The caterer is the professional provider of food and true professionalism in any field means being aware of all there is to know about one's subject.

The public are becoming more interested in nutrition. It would make sense, therefore, for the caterer to take every possible step to stay ahead of his market.

Sadly the deep-fat fryer is still one of the busiest pieces of equipment in most catering establishments.

Caterers must accept responsibility for helping to shape the nation's diet. One must ask if they are professionally equipped to do so. It is unfortunate that in the past a certain amount of antagonism existed between caterers and dietitians which did not allow the development of the liaison necessary between the two professions. Many caterers in hospitals now work closely with dietitians and the nutritional balance of hospital meals may well be reflecting increasingly the working relationship between these two.

Other caterers may still feel that they have expert knowledge of nutrition. In fact, in the UK the training of many catering managers outside the National Health Service is directed mostly towards cost control and operational efficiency, and may place nutrition as a subject of minor importance (Corr, 1979). It is possible to qualify in catering management in parts of the UK without ever having studied nutrition as a specific subject.

A carefully balanced diet in a hospital is vitally important for the care and recovery of all patients. In providing this the caterer has the opportunity of demonstrating how good nutrition can be put into practice, and, despite the widespread misconception to the contrary, there is no need for conflict between commercial interests and sound nutrition.

Pharmacists

Health education and health maintenance are part of the traditional role of the pharmacist, particularly those engaged in general practice. Such education is important if medicines are to provide maximum benefit with minimum harm.

Not only do we need pharmacists to advise on misuse of drugs and self-medication but they must also, with the increasing potency of drugs, be able to advise on any side effects. This is particularly important when dealing with the elderly who are frequent takers of drugs and can be most vulnerable nutritionally.

On the retail side, the pharmacist is constantly being asked to advise the general public on food—everything from baby foods to vitamin supplements to so-called "slimming" foods. Apart from information given by a manufacturer or its company representative, the pharmacist will not normally receive any other data on these products. Yet it is he or his shop assistant who is asked to advise on usage and suitability. Pharmacists frequently comment on their need for more comprehensive nutritional information to help them deal with this aspect of their work. Let us hope that the importance of this topic is recognized more fully when training courses are reviewed.

Nursing

Nursing is by tradition a conservative profession and although nurse education should be a fertile area for change, the effect of tradition and professional resistance can make innovation difficult.

Nurses are trained, rather than educated, to use their skills, which are in the main practical (Birchenall, 1980).

Most hospital wards still depend on student nurses as a main labour force. The learner nurse is often working in a task-orientated way, rather than a patient-orientated way, although with the introduction of "the nursing process" the emphasis is beginning to change.

It is becoming increasingly apparent that the nutritional status of all patients is an important factor in their health before, and their recovery rate after, surgery (Dickerson, 1979).

However well the catering department prepares the food, the responsibility for ensuring that the patient has an adequate nutritional intake must rest with the nursing staff on the ward. It must be the nurse's duty to inform the medical and dietetic staff if she considers that a patient's lack of appetite could be limiting the rate of recovery.

The nurse is also the person who gives guidance to relatives on the care of the patient on returning home. This will often mean giving advice on a sensible eating pattern. In most cases any modified dietary regime will have been dealt with by a dietitian, but in many areas where no such expertise is available the nurse will also have to advise patients and relatives about coping with the limitations of a modified diet at home. This is not an easy thing to do and it would appear that very rarely are nurses, through their training, equipped to deal adequately with this task.

Midwives

Midwifery as a profession is involved so closely with human hope, joy and sometimes grief that it is understandable that a midwife must at times distance herself from her clients.

The time of her involvement, however, is one when motivation can be at its greatest, thus giving her an opportunity to advise which is much envied by other educators.

The health visitor

The major role of health visitors is preventive health care. They have historically been concerned with mothers and babies but their role has now expanded to include, at least in theory, responsibility for the health education of the whole population. The potential of the health visitor in nutrition education must be realized (Fig. 3).

Most health visitors work on attachment to GPs. Routine work involves antenatal and postnatal clinics, home visits and school visits, often to teach within a health education course.

Concern has been expressed, however, about the small amount of nutrition included in training courses for health visitors. It has been stated (Wofinden, 1968) that applied nutrition is no longer stipulated as being an essential component of their training. It is felt by many that the advice the health visitor can provide on nutritional matters, therefore, can only be of a general nature, despite being the person best placed in the community to provide nutritional guidance.

Working as they do on attachment to GPs, they seem to be the ideal people to run group therapy classes, e.g. for obese patients.

Their work with school nurses could also provide useful opportunities to become involved with "active" nutrition education.

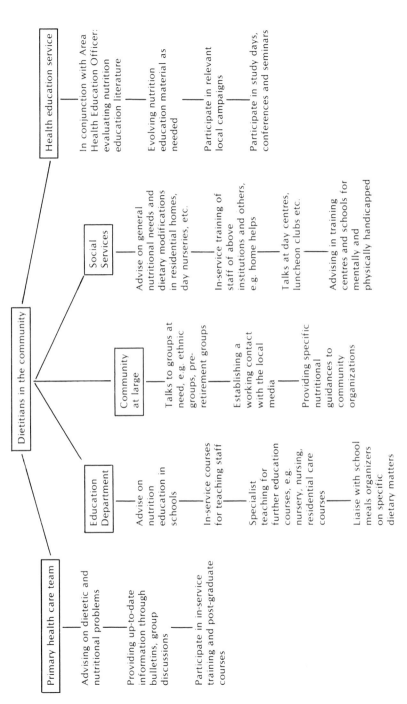

Figure 3 The role of the dietitian in the community

Dietitians in the community

Primary health care team

Advising on dietetic and nutritional problems

Providing up-to-date information through bulletins, group discussions

Participate in in-service training and post-graduate courses

Education Department

Advise on nutrition education in schools

In-service courses for teaching staff

Specialist teaching for further education courses, e.g. nursery, nursing, residential care courses

Liaise with school meals organizers on specific dietary matters

Community at large

Talks to groups at need, e.g. ethnic groups, pre-retirement groups

Establishing a working contact with the local media

Providing specific nutritional guidances to community organizations

Social Services

Advise on general nutritional needs and dietary modifications in residential homes, day nurseries, etc.

In-service training of staff of above institutions and others, e.g. home helps

Talks at day centres, luncheon clubs etc.

Advising in training centres and schools for mentally and physically handicapped

Health education service

In conjunction with Area Health Education Officer: evaluating nutrition education literature

Evolving nutrition education material as needed

Participate in relevant local campaigns

Participate in study days, conferences and seminars

Community nurses

Community nurses, like health visitors, mostly work on attachment to GPs and their responsiblity is to provide total nursing to their patients in their own homes, where they can also teach relatives about the care of the patient.

Many of our potential nutritional problems relate to the elderly or the housebound, and both of these groups are seen by the community nurse.

A visit to give an injection or change a dressing provides an ideal opportunity for the nurse to talk about food, for example, about keeping an adequate food storecupboard.

There is little about teaching in the basic training of nurses and very little time and attention is paid to it in community nurse training. Yet we know that a much higher percentage of information given in a person's own environment will be remembered, than in a more stressful hospital atmosphere. It is also likely that the information would be of a practical nature and more likely to be implemented.

The social worker

Social workers are required in all hospitals and in the community working in collaboration with the GP and the hospital doctor.

They are often the people to develop close working relationships with those in the community at greatest risk nutritionally, for example the physically disabled, the elderly or the deprived family. As a result the social worker can see the home living conditions, be aware of any financial or social constraints which may be operating. The success of any advice given to those families by other health professionals may well be dependent upon the social worker's assessment of the family's needs and limitations.

Dietitians

As we have seen, advice on nutrition can come from many professional sources. It is essential, therefore, that the advice is co-ordinated and the message given is consistent.

The need for authoritative advice is apparent. Professional staff, like many other members of the general public, consider themselves experts in nutrition, merely because they eat three meals a day. They may be tempted to give their personal opinions as a consensus view. Many health-care professionals will have trained several years ago and, as with other scientific subjects, new information about nutrition is constantly becoming available. Lack of time for reading or attending study courses could well mean that out-of-date information could be communicated.

It is vital that the community as a whole should have access to professional nutritional advice. One of the most valuable ways in which dietitians can use their expertise is in advising fellow professionals.

The reorganization of the National Health Service in 1974 provided, with a new dietetic management structure, an ideal opportunity for expansion into the community. Until that date no more than a dozen dietitians were fully employed working in the community. Now with District Dietitians given the task of managing both the hospital and community services, it has been possible to increase greatly the educational role of dietitians in the community.

Conclusion

The objective of a dietitian working in the field of nutrition education must be to promote a better understanding of nutrition and health so that the general public will have a clearer appreciation of the importance of their life-style to their health.

It is essential that the public are equipped with sufficient information to enable them to judge the value of the various messages that confront them from the media and elsewhere.

We must all ensure that the health-care professional is qualified to respond to the ever-changing needs of society. Only in this way can we ever hope to achieve a healthier future.

References

Birchenall, P. D. (1980) Innovation in Nurse Education. *Nursing Times,* **76**, Part 2, 951–9.

British Dietetic Association and Department of Health and Social Security Catering and Dietetic Branch (1977) "A Challenge to Change": a tape/slide programme based on a joint working party report. DHSS Catering and Dietetic Branch, London.

British Nutrition Foundation, Department of Health and Social Security and Health Education Council (1977) "Nutrition Education: Report of a Working Party", HMSO, London.

Corr, F. (March 1979) Nutrition—Caterers don't want to know. *Hotel and Catering Review,* 15–18.

Dickerson, J. W. T. (1979) "Nutrition in an Age of Technology". University of Surrey, Guildford.

Fieldhouse, P. (1979) What the doctor knows. *Nutrition and Food Science,* **57,** 2–3.

Rhodes, P. (1980) The framework of graduate medical education. *Lancet,* **i,** 356–9.

Wofinden, R. C. (1968) The case for, and the work of, a community dietitian. *Proceedings of the Nutrition Society,* **27,** 24.

World Health Organization First Regional Workshop on the Teaching of Nutrition in Schools of Medicine (1974).

Learning about Food within the Primary School Curriculum

Ruth Squire

Ashley Down Infant's School, Bristol

The Plowden Committee said "At the heart of the educational process lies the child" (Central Advisory Council for Education, 1966b). Teachers play a vital role in this educational process, and are concerned to do what is best for the children in their care.

We believe that the early years are of crucial importance for learning, and firm foundations must be laid for sound building in the future. We are concerned with the intellectual, social and emotional development of each child, the whole child, and we try to cater sensitively for the individual child's varying needs.

However, nutrition education is one aspect of a child's development which, I believe, is neglected. Children are regularly involved with physical education, movement and games, but many schools are not educating the "inner" child, which is so vitally important for the child's continued health and happiness.

The child's present and future depends on good health, and I believe one of the most important aims of education should be that a child develops a positive and responsible attitude to nutrition and good health. This entails developing and encouraging good eating habits from a wide and varied choice of food, encouraging the idea that good health is natural, and ensuring an awareness of the dangers of obesity and dental caries.

Nutrition education is, after all, an education for life. Attitudes develop early, and children are often capable of learning much more than we expect.

Most secondary schools now operate a cafeteria system for school meals and many children find great difficulty in making a wise selection. I did hear of one secondary school child choosing three portions of jelly for his lunch. The need to develop good eating habits and to balance meals go together. I have found it useful to let children choose their favourite meal and then discuss whether it is a sensible choice. Children can plan their food for a day.

Our message for healthy eating is based on "Eating for Health" issued by the Department of Health and Social Security (DHSS, 1978).

We stress moderation—a little of everything and not too much of anything—less sugar, less fat, more dietary fibre, and we encourage the eating of wholemeal bread. We encourage three meals a day, and say it is best not to eat between meals.

The school tuck shop which sells biscuits, whilst raising money for school funds is not, I feel, operating in the children's best interest and is, therefore, not good educational practice. Other less damaging ways can be found of raising money for school funds.

I believe that schools, as part of the community, can and should do a great deal to ensure the nutrition education of the individual. Primary schools have a very enthusiastic audience in their most receptive years, and whether nutrition education is part of the school curriculum depends primarily on the attitude of the headteacher and staff. I feel teachers need to be aware of the importance of nutrition education and good health, and be convinced of the intellectual, social and emotional value of food activities in the curriculum. Excellent illustrative materials are available for use in schools, but they are not effective without an enthusiastic teacher. Enthusiasm is infectious, and teachers have a responsibility here to enjoyably, imaginatively and sensitively emphasize nutrition education so that children see it as important.

Nursery rhymes provide valuable, rhythmic and sequential learning experiences and can be adapted to suit a particular situation—for example, there was an old woman who lived in a potato, she had so many children and they all ate potatoes, boiled, baked, roast and chips. This is an excellent opportunity to emphasize the nutritional value of eating potatoes, and to stress moderation in the consumption of chips.

How can effective nutrition education be achieved in primary schools? Primary teachers are not home economists or dietitians, and there are polymathic demands on their time.

Initial training, and in-service education and training (i.e. the continuation of professional development) both have their part to play. The good teacher is always learning and in-service education and training is vital for teacher development and support. Also necessary is the exchange of expertise and skills between the teachers themselves.

Within the County of Avon there is an agreed need, felt by all concerned with the education of children, that the promotion of nutrition education and food activities in the primary school curriculum is an essential and vital development, and appropriate courses are provided for teachers involving practical work and curriculum development. Continuity is essential in all areas of the curriculum, and effective co-operation and understanding is being activated between secondary school home economists and primary school teachers. Valuable help and support is given to teachers by the Local Education Authority advisers, and particularly by those with particular responsibility for this area of the curriculum. Effective help and information is also available to schools from the Area Health Authority education officer for nutrition and from community dietitians.

Co-operation and partnership between the different providers is essential and is so beneficial for the children.

In his book "When Children Learn", David Boorer (1974) says "the art of teaching is the art of motivating". There is no doubt that if children are interested and motivated, they will persevere to acquire new techniques and skills.

Children are interested to hear that Queen Elizabeth the First had bad black teeth, and that this was attributed, by a German visitor to her court, to the English defect of eating too much sugar (Davidson *et al.,* 1972).

They are fascinated to hear from the keeper at the zoo that Henry the orang-utan had suffered from bad headaches, and he kept holding his head in his hands. One day Henry opened his mouth and the keeper saw a bad, broken tooth and he realized that Henry was in agony from toothache. Children are keen to read the list of ingredients on cereal packets to find out if sugar has already been added—if so, they do not need to add any more.

Counting teeth is a useful and pertinent mathematical activity. Claire, aged 6 years, wrote "Mummy has 30 teeth in her mouth and 2 in a box, because she had them taken out, 16 at the top and 14 at the bottom".

A group of 10- and 11-year-old girls made up their own teeth dance. They chose the music, and arranged the percussion accompaniment. They also made their own costumes and effects, and so reinforced their learning in a very meaningful and enjoyable way.

Children enjoy experiments using disclosing tablets and are interested in different teeth.

I am convinced that many children who underperform in school do not always lack ability. They often lack interest and motivation, and a belief in the possibility of success.

Self-motivation only results from a child's interest and worthwhile activities. There is no doubt that children do enjoy food activities, and I have yet to encounter any problems with lack of motivation in this area of the curriculum.

Food is warmth, love and security. Nutrition education goes on in the classroom and involves much oral work and discussion—often with children sitting on a carpet near the teacher. There is close contact and the overall atmosphere helps build up secure relationships between the children and teachers. The group situation in food activities is very beneficial for all children, and especially for junior children with learning difficulties, who receive extra adult attention and more practice in basic skills. They then have the opportunity to understand the processes which they had probably not understood in the classroom, and, most important, they are not made to feel "different".

Food activities are a means of making nutrition education meaningful and enjoyable, as well as providing interesting and pleasant ways of learning. Both can be successfully integrated into the primary school curriculum, and are a vital part of the wider curriculum.

Many disciplines and skills are involved in food activities; as well as manipulative skills, there is counting, estimating, ordering, measuring, timing, making graphs, modelling, painting, reading and writing. One needs to be able to read the recipe; this is meaningful language development and provides a valuable sequencing activity.

Work cards are provided for use with each recipe and are graded to suit all age levels and abilities in the primary school.

Food activities also encourage good creative writing.

Aristotle said "Nothing is in the mind which was not first in the senses". There is no doubt that all primary children do need and benefit from valuable sensory experiences; for example, when making bread, dough is sticky and pliable. This is meaningful language development and aids concept learning.

I remember Philippa kneading the dough and saying "it's all yummy and squashy"— can you remember the satisfying, soothing feeling that one gets from such an activity?—and Stephen saying "it's hard work".

We no longer support "the rucksack view of knowledge of the old elementary schools" (Dearden, 1968), but there is no doubt that the basic skills, the 3 Rs, must be effectively taught and learned. We do need planned programmes for the basic skills; for example, there must be a definite progression in mathematics.

Food activities can be an effective "coat-hanger" for basic skills, a way of enjoyably and usefully applying knowledge and skills.

If basic skills are taught in isolation the child can become bored and learning meaningless. It is interesting to note that in the latest survey of Primary Education in England by H.M. Inspectors, it was found that 9- and 11-year-old children who had been taught in the wider curriculum, performed better in the National Foundation for Education Research's standardized tests than those who had been taught basic skills in isolation (Department of Education and Science, 1978).

Cooking aids scientific concept development—the ingredients change when they are cooked—can this change be reversed?

Children are encouraged to develop logical and enquiring minds and, as Mollie Brearley says in her book "Fundamentals in the First School", "building up the power to think clearly and effectively, should be the constant aim of teachers" (Brearley, 1969).

All areas of the curriculum are important. For example, a child should know about the past and develop an historical awareness. I heard of one little boy who went to London and told his teacher that he had fed the pigeons in "Travolta Square".

A project or topic work is a natural and effective way of integrating all areas of the curriculum. The Plowden Committee advocated project work as a means of breaking down rigid subject barriers, and recommended flexibility in the curriculum (Central Advisory Council for Education, 1966a).

I believe nutrition education and food activities could and should be included naturally in all projects, as a vital and important area of the curriculum, together with language development, science, music, mathematics, creative activities and so on. I remember a few years ago a teacher said to me, "I did nutrition last term", but nutrition education should not be dealt with in isolation, or dealt with once and then forgotten about. To achieve lasting and effective results nutrition education needs to be on-going and incorporated into many and varied projects.

Sometimes in schools "cooking" is a separate activity, and there is no connection between the food being prepared and learning going on in the classroom. If there is any connection it is incidental and haphazard, and good eating habits are not discussed.

Usually these teachers, parents and children are suffering from the "fancy cakes syndrome". I remember a young student teacher once saying to me that she thought making an open sandwich was too easy for junior age children, and could they make rock cakes instead!

Topic diagrams and flow charts are very useful for integrating all areas of the curriculum. It is a planned preparation, an ordering of the teachers ideas, yet allows for flexibility to cater for childrens' ideas and interests.

As Ieuan Lloyd says in his article "The integrated day in the primary school", "we can fan the spark that comes from the child but the teacher must often do some flamethrowing" (Lloyd, 1971).

The important point is that if teachers are aware of the learning possibilities in food activities they can plan their development to the children's advantage.

An activity like making cheese biscuits needs to be thought out. To structure and plan the integration of all areas of the curriculum is very demanding of the teacher's time, energy and skill, but it is infinitely more rewarding. It is sometimes surprising how much an activity, such as making cheese biscuits, can be extended and learning developed.

Food activities can be the start of a project, for example about the

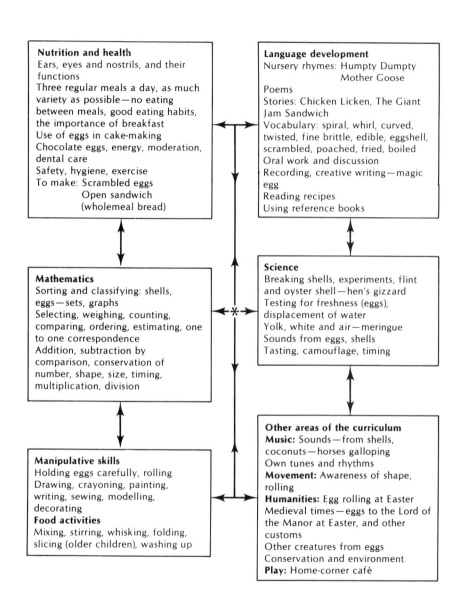

Nutrition and health
Ears, eyes and nostrils, and their functions
Three regular meals a day, as much variety as possible—no eating between meals, good eating habits, the importance of breakfast
Use of eggs in cake-making
Chocolate eggs, energy, moderation, dental care
Safety, hygiene, exercise
To make: Scrambled eggs
            Open sandwich
            (wholemeal bread)

Language development
Nursery rhymes: Humpty Dumpty
                           Mother Goose
Poems
Stories: Chicken Licken, The Giant Jam Sandwich
Vocabulary: spiral, whirl, curved, twisted, fine brittle, edible, eggshell, scrambled, poached, fried, boiled
Oral work and discussion
Recording, creative writing—magic egg
Reading recipes
Using reference books

Mathematics
Sorting and classifying: shells, eggs—sets, graphs
Selecting, weighing, counting, comparing, ordering, estimating, one to one correspondence
Addition, subtraction by comparison, conservation of number, shape, size, timing, multiplication, division

Science
Breaking shells, experiments, flint and oyster shell—hen's gizzard
Testing for freshness (eggs), displacement of water
Yolk, white and air—meringue
Sounds from eggs, shells
Tasting, camouflage, timing

Manipulative skills
Holding eggs carefully, rolling
Drawing, crayoning, painting, writing, sewing, modelling, decorating
Food activities
Mixing, stirring, whisking, folding, slicing (older children), washing up

Other areas of the curriculum
Music: Sounds—from shells, coconuts—horses galloping
Own tunes and rhythms
Movement: Awareness of shape, rolling
Humanities: Egg rolling at Easter
Medieval times—eggs to the Lord of the Manor at Easter, and other customs
Other creatures from eggs
Conservation and environment
Play: Home-corner café

Figure 1 The integrated curriculum: planned and structured learning which could develop from the starting point * SHELLS. (From *Food for Learning* by Ruth Squires to be published by Forbes Publications Ltd.)

apple harvest, but they can also be integrated into projects developing from other starting points, for example, *glass* or *shells* (Fig. 1).

It is valuable social education for children to know and appreciate that there are many different foods in the world, all providing a balanced diet for healthy living, in different cultures and climes. A Caribbean project developed as a result of trying out Caribbean recipes in my school, where approximately 5% of the children are of West Indian and Asian origin; we had the support and help of the Multi-Cultural Education Centre.

I feel such work is essential to prepare children for life in a multi-cultural society and to promote effective understanding and racial harmony.

Nutrition education can be integrated into many activities, and learning extended by informed adult involvement. In one classroom the home corner was turned into a pirate ship and there was much meaningful play and discussion. The teacher was a visiting pirate, and she extended the children's learning by her initiation, intervention and participation.

I firmly believe that the education of children should be a "partnership" between parents and teachers. Research has shown how important are the pre-school years, and the continuing influence of the home and parental encouragement throughout the child's school life (Bynner, 1972).

Food activities are a useful means of involving parents in school, and also for extending nutrition education to the "whole family" (Central Advisory Council for Education, 1966c).

Involvement in school helps parents to understand how children learn; the need for practical work and understanding; the group situation; the integrated curriculum; and essential adult involvement. It helps parents to understand how their own children are learning, and makes them aware of the ways in which they can help support them.

It is important that parents are asked to do only tasks of which they are capable so that they can feel they are needed and doing a worthwhile job. I have regular meetings with the parents involved in food activities, and it is surprising how much useful information can be diplomatically imparted over a friendly cup of tea.

Food activities help parents to become aware of the need for a wide and varied choice of foods, and eating for health. This is particularly important in these days of rising prices, when smaller numbers of children are having school meals and a greater proportion of children are bringing sandwiches to eat at lunchtime.

It is pleasing that many of our families are now eating wholemeal bread, not adding sugar to cereals, eating fresh fruit and appreciating why we do not sell biscuits in school. It will be interesting to see if we can develop the school as a community catalyst with the Education and the Health Authorities working together, and extend our nutrition education further to all age groups in the area community.

The onus for parental involvement rests with the school and food activities are a useful means of involving parents, and utilizing their skill and expertise. Varied and informed adult involvement is important in motivating children to learn. I remember a parent at one of our assemblies was a dental hygienist and she volunteered to come into school and work with groups of children. Both children and staff benefited from this involvement.

The health visitor also comes into school as part of our team, and works with all groups of children, reinforcing and extending the learning which has gone on in the classroom. This is particularly important with regard to children with weight problems; nutrition education is for all, and no child is singled out and made to feel "different".

Continuity is important in all areas of the curriculum and, hopefully, children who have been taught in the integrated wider curriculum will not "compartmentalize" their learning but will be able to question, reason, be adaptable, and apply their knowledge and skills to many and varied situations.

Food activities can provide a continuity of learning experiences between the different provisions in education, and primary school teachers can lay the firm foundations of nutrition education. The specialist teachers in secondary schools can build on those foundations; there will be study in greater depth, and nutrition education will be effective and lasting.

The children of today are very soon the parents of tomorrow. Schools can influence present-day habits, and can do much to influence future behaviour and attitudes, and so help to lay the foundations of a happy, healthy and caring society.

Author's note: This paper relates to the contents of my book "Food for Learning" to be published by Forbes Publications.

References

Boorer, David (1974) "When Children Learn". Evans, London

Brearley, M. (1969) "Fundamentals in the First School". Basil Blackwell, Oxford.

Bynner, J. M. (1972) "Parents' Attitudes to Education". HMSO, London

Central Advisory Council for Education (1966a) "Children and their Primary Schools", Vol. 1. HMSO, London.

Central Advisory Council for Education (1966b) "Children and their Primary Schools", Vol. 1, Chap. 2, para. 9. HMSO, London.

Central Advisory Council for Education (1966c) "Childen and their Primary Schools", Vol. 1, Chap. 4, para. 129. HMSO, London.

Davidson, Sir Stanley, Passmore, R. and Brock, J. F. (1972) "Human Nutrition and Dietetics". Churchill Livingstone, Edinburgh.

Dearden, R. F. (1968) "The Philosophy of Primary Education". Routledge and Kegan Paul, London.

The Department of Health and Social Security (1978) "Eating for Health". HMSO, London.

The Department of Education and Science (1978) "Primary Education in England", a survey by HM inspector of Schools, Chap. 8, para 8. HMSO, London.

Lloyd, Ieuan (1971) The integrated day in the primary school. *In* "The Integrated Day in Theory and Practice", (Walton, J., ed.). Ward Lock Educational, London.

Nutrition and the Media

Tony Smith

British Medical Journal, London

When I was first asked to talk about nutrition and the media I saw my task as easy enough. What I planned to do was to spend a month or so looking at newspapers, television, radio, bookstalls and publishers' lists for articles, programmes and books dealing with nutrition. What I found was rather different from my expectations. These sources give an enormous amount of attention to food and drink—but they refer to the nutritional implications much less often. The message is mainly: eat (or drink) this and you will enjoy it, or be happy, or be seen to be successful, or beautiful, or sexually attractive: only very seldom is there any implication that the product will improve your health.

And when the message does contain explicit nutritional comment, depressingly often the content is either false or nonsensical. As an example, the label on a packet of mung beans, sold by an old-established firm of English seed merchants, reads:

> "a new instant vegetable, sweet and full of flavour, and loaded with health giving nutrients including vitamin E. Doctors now consider vitamin E absolutely essential to the body and have concluded that its use is one of the great medical discoveries of the century. It can reverse as well as prevent the symptoms of the ageing process. It acts as a vasodilator, i.e. allows more blood to flow through constricted arteries and veins and improves bad circulation in arterial plaques. Recently the Soviet Academy of Medical Sciences and Nutritional Institute have found that sufficient vitamin E gives a definite boost to the performance of athletes. And it has been demonstrated in laboratory and clinical studies that vitamin E is effective against a multitude of diseases."

More often, of course, misinformation of this kind comes in the form of a book or magazine article—but I shall come to those later. And I hasten to add that my month-long surveillance of publications yielded many examples of accurate, educative, accounts of dietetics and food science, nutritional, basics and material suitable for A-level students. But few of these excellent publications were even aimed at a mass audience—let alone likely to reach that target.

Why emphasize the mass audience, you may ask? The answer—at least in a medical context—is plain enough. In many common diseases from heart disease to stomach cancer; in perinatal mortality; and in simple measures of nutritional health such as growth rates in childhood; social classes IV and V fare worse than do skilled workers and the professional classes. In some cases there is clear evidence and in others suggestive evidence that these variations are due to class differences in diet. If changes are to be made in our eating habits as a nation, the most urgent need is for change in the popular, mass diet rather than in middle-class fashions.

So what influences the way people eat—most people, that is, not the middle classes with their minority groups who for most of this century pursued vegetarian asceticism in their open-toed sandals? People choose what they eat as a result of a whole panoply of pressures and persuasions. Cultural background and parental example provide the baseline, but people—and especially the young—also pick up ideas from friends and neighbours, local restaurants, and foreign travel. Today, however, we are concerned with the more direct and commercial pressures: advertisements on television, in magazines and newspapers and food journals; radio programmes, articles in the papers, and accounts on television and in books and magazines.

No one would claim that advertisers are much interested in nutrition. Their job is to sell products, from chocolate bars to instant TV dinners, and they do so by techniques that rely heavily on instant gratification rather than on any promotion of the long-term effects of the food or drink. The content of this advertising of food and drink came as a surprise to me when I started to record it. On television, in newspapers, and in magazines the dominant products are alcoholic drinks, promoted with great skill and often in visually very appealing terms. On most evenings television viewing from 4 pm to midnight showed, first of all, an hour or so of sweet drinks and chocolate bars, peanuts and crisps directed at children; but as soon as peak viewing time began the dominant products were beers, vermouths and vodkas.

Study of magazines, newspapers and hoardings shows a similar pattern: drinks come top of the list—with soft drinks competing for attention with alcohol, and a lot of promotion for various brands of instant coffee; next come chocolate bars and sweets; and other snacks such as peanuts and crisps. Clearly the advertising agencies would like to see the population sitting in front of their television sets, munching snack foods and drinking either sugary or alcoholic drinks, between frenetic visits to supermarkets and discount warehouses.

Next I turned to articles on cooking—the regular columns in newspapers, the features in magazines, books and journals. You will all be familiar with the content of this type of journalism: it follows the year round, with an emphasis on eggs at Easter, strawberries in June, salads in the summer and even goose at Michaelmas. All too often, regrettably enough, the meals suggested contain a series of dishes that would have challenged even Gargantua's appetites. Sometimes they seem to be chosen for their visual appeal—no bad thing when seeking to tempt a jaded appetite, but the target is rarely the invalid and more often the sated gourmand. Most cookery journalism makes no reference to nutrition. Perhaps the expert cooks are all too well aware of the high fat content of their sauces, the excess of sugar in their elaborate puddings and indeed the appalling richness of so much gourmet food.

Sometimes a throw-away line or two will refer to some nutritional qualities of the ingredients of a particular dish: few cooks seem able to talk about spinach without using words such as "nutritious" or "health-giving", and making some reference to iron as an essential ingredient of the diet. No doubt the cult of spinach can be traced back to Popeye the sailorman and even earlier: it is a splendid example of the popular belief that if the diet needs to contain some trace element or vitamin then the more it contains the better it must be.

Most cookery journalism, then, is outside the range of this paper. But there are several important exceptions. First comes the whole slimming industry—the diets designed for readers who want to lose weight. Here the emphasis is on peeling off the pounds rather than cleaning out the arteries, but very often the result is excellent in nutritional terms. In fairness to the slimming experts, I must say that the diets they recommend nowadays mostly seem more reasonable than the crash programmes that were so popular a few years back. The current advocates of total fasting seem to emphasize its mind-enhancing effects as much as its use as a means of losing weight fast. Leaving them aside, there is now much less of the orange juice and black coffee nonsense and more attempt to produce balanced diets of 1000—1200 calories which can be sustained for long periods.

The second exception to the corrupting influence of cookery journalism is the group of diets specifically designed to reduce the risks of heart disease. Enough people are now aware of the importance of the world-wide epidemic of coronary artery disease for there to be a ready audience for accounts of diets designed to reduce the amounts of cholesterol and low-density lipoproteins in the blood. A recent example is a cookery book produced by Professor Barry Lewis and his wife "The Heart Book. Living Well and Taking Care of Your Heart".

My anxiety here is that the target of these publications still seems to be the middle-class, middle brow or intellectual, who reads quality newspapers and listens to BBC Radio 4 and so has heard and absorbed the message already. Little mention of the *cuisine minceur* appears in the mass-readership newspapers.

What seems to be lacking in most cookery journalism is any recognition by the authors that there is, in fact, a reasonable consensus on what constitutes a medically prudent diet—one containing less fat and less refined carbohydrate, and more cereals and vegetables than the recent tradition in affluent society both in north-west Europe and the USA. What a pity more emphasis is not given to the nutritional soundness of the southern European diet based on olive oil; after all, it proves popular enough with many of the British tourists who flock to the Mediterranean during the summer months.

Instead—and this is my main criticism of the way journalists handle nutrition—publicity is given to faddish fashionable theories linking diet and disease with little apparent concern for the quantity or quality of the evidence behind them. When Bruce Page, now editor of the New Statesman, was heading the Insight team at the Sunday Times he used to say there were only two news stories: "we name the guilty man" and "arrow points to faulty part". All too often, news items and features about food and nutrition fall into the second category: the nub of the story is that some food is the previously unsuspected cause of a common disease.

As an example, look at the enthusiasm with which the new media seized on the series of reports linking artificial sweeteners—first cyclamates and later saccharine—with bladder cancer in rats. This was a marvellous "doom-watch" topic: almost everyone must at some time have taken some saccharine or cyclamate in a soft drink, so every potential reader or television viewer would have grounds for personal concern. Now in many cases the immediate cover given to the news was reasonably balanced, pointing out the frequency of bladder tumours in rats and the dangers of extrapolating from animals to man—but the seeds of doubt were sown.

However, subsequent careful studies in man—such as Sir Richard Doll's examination of the frequency of bladder cancer in diabetics and in the rest of the population—showed no evidence linking human bladder cancer with artificial sweeteners. Yet when these studies virtually cleared these compounds of any danger to man, these negative reports received little publicity. "Not-guilty" verdicts against foods and additives do not seem to be news.

Indeed I wonder what the cumulative effect of these doom-watch stories must be. Another example is the link between cancer of the large bowel and diet. The considerable geographical variations in the incidence of this type of cancer suggests an environmental cause, and at various times in recent years associations have been reported between colonic cancer and the fat content of the diet, or the amount of meat, or the consumption of beer. These are, of course, no more than associations: what they mean remains far from clear. But they make marvellous shock-horror stories for the

Sunday papers—guaranteed to rivet the attention of any reader after a lunch of roast beef washed down with a few pints of bitter.

The currently fashionable theory of this kind is that many unexplained major illnesses, from rheumatoid arthritis to schizophrenia, not to mention a host of minor symptoms from headache to fatigue, are due to food allergy. Again this is a marvellously compelling idea for the public at large. It trades on their vague suspicions that modern food is not as wholesome as old fashioned "natural" products with the suggestion by many food allergists that the essential culprits are additives, preservatives and flavouring agents. Other targets are coffee and tea and chickens (perhaps only battery chickens).

Now there may be a few individuals who are truly allergic to one or more foods, and occasionally a patient is seen with quite specific symptoms attributable to the amount of coffee he drinks. But I believe there is little convincing evidence that any substantial numbers of sick people are suffering from the effects of specific food allergies when the exponents of that theory can provide no clear explanation of the mechanism, nor indeed any consistent pattern, of symptoms.

About five years ago the national papers—or some of them—took up with great enthusiasm the suggestion that the puzzling, crippling nerve disorder multiple sclerosis was in some way attributable to a hypersensitivity to gluten, the protein in wheat. Now gluten sensitivity is already known to be the basis of coeliac disease, an uncommon but serious disorder which, if untreated, stunts growth and causes chronic invalidism in childhood. Children—and adults, who are affected less often—with coeliac disease can be returned to normal health dramatically and gratifyingly by providing them with a diet that contains no gluten. So when a few enthusiasts began to claim that a gluten-free diet was also effective in multiple sclerosis, they found a ready audience.

Cynical old journalists such as myself have lost count of the numbers of new "cures" for multiple sclerosis that have been publicized only to be covered by the sands of time. The disease causes false hopes and heartbreaks because of the extraordinary, quite unique capacity of sufferers to make sustained remissions. Not all that rarely, someone who has been confined to a wheelchair, with slurred speech and partial vision, can be restored to normal or near health within a week or two. Sadly, all too often, such a recovery is only temporary, but it may be sustained for many years or indeed permanently. Naturally enough, in such cases all concerned look for some explanation—and if, as is almost inevitable, some new treatment was being tried at the time, it is given the credit for recovery. So there is difficulty in finding a few dramatic case histories to bolster almost any proposed new treatment for multiple sclerosis.

In the case of the gluten-free diet, the campaign by its supporters was sustained and at times very aggressive. The Department of Health came under heavy criticism for denying the treatment to NHS patients. No one listened to neurologists who doubted the theory and questioned the evidence on which it was based: in the end the Multiple Sclerosis Society was put under such pressure that it set up a trial of the treatment. The result was negative. No difference could be detected in the progress of the disease in patients on the diet and those eating normal food.

I would like to make two more points about that episode. Firstly, a gluten-free diet is very restrictive, not to say monotonous. To inflict it, without good evidence, on patients desperate for any remedy for their disease seems to me to be heartless irresponsibility. Secondly, despite the clear proof that it does not work, a few enthusiasts can still be found propagandizing its virtues. That obstinacy illustrates one of the features of the strange land of make believe in which so many food-faddists live: the medical establishment can never convince them they are wrong. I can understand that attitude in a North American setting, where doctors can always be attacked on the grounds that their high financial rewards depend on their discrediting all forms of alternative medicine. Here in Britain I think the medical establishment is more receptive to alternative techniques. It has, for example, been reasonably receptive to the use of meditation for the treatment of high blood pressure or of acupuncture for the relief of some forms of chronic pain.

But I am straying away from my theme. Gluten and multiple sclerosis is one example of the media giving premature, unwarranted publicity to a magic cure for one of the failures of orthodox medicine. There are many others. By far the most persistent is the belief that vitamin C cures not only the common cold but also many other disorders: schizophrenia is also alleged to be a vitamin deficiency; and the relentless progress of senile dementia is said simply to be a manifestation of chronic deficiency of the B vitamins. In all of these cases the presentation is along similar lines. Firstly, the failure of orthodox medicine is catalogued, with gloomy statistics of the frequency of the disease. Secondly, some more or less eminent scientist is named as the originator of the treatment; and thirdly, the medical establishment is castigated for its failure to acknowledge the outstanding benefits of the treatment.

Now I can imagine that some of you are saying that I am a typically arrogant doctor myself, refusing to listen to unorthodox theories simply because they are unorthodox. My answer is simple enough: when evidence is good enough any treatment will be incorporated into orthodox medicine. If I look at three of the most common diseases for which "cures" are given publicity—cancer, multiple sclerosis and mental handicap in children—I can list scores of claims but none that have proved effective. Doctors do not ignore unorthodox cures simply because they are unorthodox. We ignore them because they do not work.

However, such black and white judgements are less easy when the claims made for a dietary modification are based at least in part on sound evidence. Perhaps the greatest turn around in medical views on diet and disease has been the case of diverticular disease. When I was a student the orthodox treatment for symptoms attributable to diverticular disease was a low residue diet—steamed fish, sieved vegetables, purées and milk puddings. Then Mr Denis Burkitt, Captain Cleave and others argued the case for increasing the fibre content of the western diet to restore bowel actions to a more normal consistency and frequency, and Mr Neil Painter showed that the addition of miller's bran to the diet relieved the symptoms of diverticular disease. Before long—and an example, if I may say so, of the way that a good new dietary treatment will be accepted even by conservative physicians—the high fibre diet had replaced the low residue diet as the mainstay of treatment for several disorders of the large bowel.

For the enthusiasts, however, that was not enough. Cleave and others have argued that the excess of refined sugar and the lack of fibre in the western diet are the causes of a whole range of diseases of civilization—from varicose veins to diabetes and peptic ulcer. Such a belief seems to reflect another characteristic of so much dietary evangelism: not satisfied with a claim that some change to our diet can relieve or prevent a particular disease, the evangelists go on to claim that they hold the secret to guaranteed good health.

Such a belief has, indeed, permeated the whole of our society in the form of the aphorism that "natural food is good for you". How many writers and commentators on food assume, at least tacitly, that food grown without chemical fertilizers and pesticides, and especially nature foods such as honey and wholemeal bread, have some intrinsic health-promoting qualities absent from the food on supermarket shelves? How many of us here today share that belief—at least to some extent?

The basis for this belief seems to me partly to be the Arcadian myth—that all life was healthier in some mythical past when the population lived in idyllic, small farming communities—and partly the conviction of so many contemporary journalists that industry, science and multinational companies are intrinsically bad, while small, ecologically caring units are necessarily good. Whatever the underlying causes, that emotional feeling is very evident. I know I believe that food from my own garden is in some way better—and I justify that belief by subjective standards such as taste and flavour. In fact, as we must all acknowledge, there is no evidence at all that, when eaten in a normal diet, so-called natural food has any advantages over that available from the supermarket: the vitamins, trace elements and other necessities for health are present in excess in the typical British diet, whatever its source, provided it contains enough variety. Subsistence on bread and butter and tea will eventually lead to scurvy no matter how home-made the bread.

I have spent most of my time listing the common faults of journalism in the field of nutrition and health. To summarize these faults: I believe journalists are too ready to give publicity to cranky, unorthodox ideas or to concepts that conform to their own prejudices— especially anti-medical, anti-chemical, anti-industrial prejudices. But it would be unfair to my colleagues to suggest that most of them are irresponsible or careless in the way they present news and features. The root cause of much of the difficulty is the attitude that our society has developed to what is and is not news. In addition to the Sunday Times' "guilty men" and "defective part" stories, our third perennial favourite is "experts disagree". Television and radio producers like nothing better than to find two spokespersons, expert or not, who can be persuaded to battle out their differences in public. So when a potential news item is offered to an editor or producer his first reaction is generally "is it controversial?" Then he may ask "is it new?" Only thirdly, and not necessarily at all, will he ask "is it true?" That is not his job, he will explain: if Nobel prizewinner A or university professor B makes a statement on a matter of public interest, that fact is itself news. And if orthodox scientific opinion rejects the so-called expert's assertion, then that makes the issue controversial, so justifying wider coverage. How often do we read or hear the newscaster say "controversy continues over the speech last week by so and so...", implying not that something has been said that might be a substantial advance on knowledge, but that something was said that was so outrageous that the scientific establishment is still simmering.

The effect of this attitude is that science journalists soon find that their balanced accounts of current concerns have less success that their reporting of extremist views. This approach is more common in popular journalism than in serious weeklies, but sensationalism of a kind is now to be found in all types of journalism. *In my view the long-term solution lies in better education for the whole population in scientific methods, so that a healthy scepticism will become more common.* As things are, I believe it would be quite easy to get publicity for a claim that the earth is in fact flat and that the experts are wrong—provided that the spokesman for the Flat Earth Society spoke well, sounded plausible, and in journalistic terms "came across well". At present those are the characteristics that lead to public attention—not the content of the message.

The Role of the Food Manufacturing Industry in Nutrition Education

Tim Fortescue

Food and Drink Industries Council, London

Manufacturing industry plays many roles on the stage of our times. It is at once the converter of raw materials; the provider of employment; the creator of wealth; the initiator of scientific research; the contributor to the Exchequer; the supporter of good causes; and a hundred more. The food manufacturing industry plays all these parts and, like any other sector, also has its own minor roles incidental to the essential nature of its operations. Thus, just as a shoe manufacturer will be interested in the techniques of the tannery, so will the food firm play its part in the better production of peas or pigs; and just as a furniture manufacturer looks to changes in living patterns, so do food processors keep a close watch on, or even seek to influence, eating patterns. Upstream of every manufacturer there are suppliers, and downstream there are customers; the manufacturer's roles inevitably include relationships with them as well as with the work-force, the share-holders, the government and the public at large.

It is not, generally speaking, the role of manufacturing industry to seek to improve the health of the general public, or to shoulder the responsibility of ensuring that people live better, or live longer, or lead healthier lives, or behave in a social rather than an anti-social way. Provided that a firm's products are not intrinsically unsafe, and its manufacturing processes neither noxious nor otherwise objectionable to an unacceptable degree, there is by and large no restriction on what it can put on the market. Governments are, however, quick to seize upon potentially dangerous goods and to legislate so that they may not be marketed except under special conditions and restrictions. Products likely to be attractive to children are especially scrutinized, and there are strict rules to govern, for instance, the materials which may be used in the manufacture of toys, especially those for infants which so readily find their way into toothless mouths. The restriction is sometimes on the retailer — fireworks, cigarettes and alcohol may not be sold to anybody under age; or even on the customer—cars and

215

guns need licences; but, for the most part, the role of the manufacturer is to put goods on the market as they are made and to sell them to whomever will buy them. The old legal principle of *caveat emptor* still pervades most transactions in most people's experience.

Special position of food

In many people's minds, food, and thus the manufacture and processing of food, is in a special category, since food, together with water and air, is an essential of life and the only one which reaches the individual through normal commercial channels. Its manufacture is thus more regulated, more open to inspection, more subject to official sampling and analysis at every stage of its journey through the processing plant than any other category of product. The most stringent checks and precautions ensure not only that the product which reaches the supermarket shelves is safe and wholesome, but also that it is "of the nature, substance and quality demanded", to quote the relevant legislation (Food and Drugs Act, 1955). The controls do not apply only to the product itself. The packaging materials must also be in accordance with the law, and the rules about food labelling, now supplemented by two European Directives (77/94/EEC and 79/112/EEC) which have been several years in the making, become more intricate every year. Every label must of course bear the name and address of the manufacturer, packer or seller, so that the blame and responsibility for any fault or damage may at once be accurately placed.

It is interesting to note that the multifarious and detailed regulations covering the manufacture and processing of food do not apply to the one-quarter of our diet which reaches our tables without first passing through the hands of a food firm. The customer can buy a cauliflower from a greengrocer, a joint of meat from a butcher or a pound of apples from a fruiterer without knowing or being able to know their source, the pesticides or hormones used by the farmer who grew or raised them, the chemicals used to preserve them on the way to market or the conditions to which they have been exposed without the protection of packaging while waiting to be sold. It is as if there existed in the minds of the public and the legislators a belief in the magical qualities of so-called "natural" food, meaning foodstuffs which have not been processed industrially, and in their absolute safety no matter what methods have been used or neglected to grow, stimulate, protect or preserve them. The customers receive and demand no information provided that they can believe that the food they buy is "fresh"; they are not convinced that frozen peas are fresher than the peas in the pod which they buy at the greengrocer, nor that the flavour they like in the fish they buy at the fishmonger is largely due to bacterial deterioration which has not taken place in frozen fish. But the frozen product must be checked, inspected and officially supervised at every point in its progress, whereas the pseudo-fresh is subject to no control at all.

Nevertheless, the food manufacturing industry welcomes the extremely close regulation of its affairs, and is close to being proud of its status as the most regimented industry of all. It is as if food companies were engaged continously in meeting and overcoming a challenge imposed upon them from the outside which makes their success—both as industrialists and technicians—all the more satisfying. The hoops on the croquet lawn are constantly being increased in number, moved and made narrower and the winners of the game are thus acknowledged as the masters of their craft. But, more seriously, the food manufacturers like to be able to lean on the strictness of the law to rebut the perennial prejudice-inspired accusations and criticisms of their industry which seem to stem from an innate, almost atavistic, conviction that it is morally and socially wrong to make a profit from food.

The war-time conditions in which nearly everybody could, in theory, buy only the basic ration at a controlled price so that there was equality of monotony are often spoken of with nostalgia and regret. Some of this reaction is undoubtedly due to the feeling that at least in those days nobody was "making money" out of food, and the corresponding feeling that nobody was able to eat more or better than anybody else. Even today, we receive complaints that a branded product is being sold at different prices in different shops and the explanation that this is a facet of competition clearly fails to satisfy. The fact that unless food production, processing and distribution were profitable, the shelves would remain as bare as they were in war-time, with all the attendant controls and black markets, seems not to occur to the critics and complainers who benefit from and enjoy as much as anybody the ever-growing variety of food now at the daily disposal of us all.

Without profit there would be no food manufacturing industry, and without sales there would be no profit. Food manufacturers must employ every technique of salesmanship if they are to stay in business, the more so because their wares are items of daily purchase and their success depends more than most on winning the loyalty of the customer to their brands. This requires not only the establishment of a reputation for high and consistent quality, but ensuring that their names and brand names are so familiar to the customers that they automatically look for them on the shelves. Continual advertising and memorable labelling are the manufacturer's chief tools.

Information through labelling

Here we arrive at the question of the provision of information to the public. The starting point must be that all advertising, labelling, and information of any sort about a product must, in the words of the Code of Conduct of the Advertising Standards Authority, be "legal, truthful, honest and decent". This should not need saying, but the code is both welcomed by the food industry and strictly followed. Labels are a form of advertising and follow the same code; but, as we have seen, food labels are also regulated in detail by national and European legislation to ensure that customers, by reference to the label, can inform themselves fully as to the composition of any product. Gradually this requirement has become, and is becoming, more refined. At first thought it would seem that to compile a list of ingredients would be a comparatively simple matter, and to print such a list on a label would tell the consumers all they wanted to know. This practice is indeed sufficient in answering one of the arguments for ingredient listing, which is that people with food allergies must be able to know from the label of a processed food that it is free from any specific ingredient. A negative statement saying that the package or can "contains no X" is not enough, since the number of items to which small minorities are allergic is so large as to be undefined. Thus to protect a very few people—or rather to enable them to protect themselves—full ingredient listing is demanded, whether or not it is of any interest to the great majority.

In the latest European Directive, an ingredient is defined as meaning any substance used in the preparation of a food which is still present at the time of sale, and the constituents of a compound ingredient must normally be given in a list of ingredients. There are rules as to the terminology to be used in describing food additives on a label and there are a number of exceptions to the basic rules. By and large, however, the consumer has the legal right to know, and the manufacturer has a statutory duty to state, what a can or package of food contains; and the information must be so set out as not to be misleading. For instance, ingredients must be listed in descending order by weight, and the label must not place special emphasis on the presence of an ingredient unless the percentage of that ingredient is declared.

These and other regulations will amply provide the customers, through food labels, with factual information about the composition of the processed foods they buy. In the great majority of cases there is no requirement for the manufacturers to give more information about any special qualities a food may have, but if they do so, they will be subject to very strict rules. If for instance, they wish to claim that a food is "suitable for fulfilling the particular nutritional requirements'' of various classes of persons, they may not do so under the proposed new labelling of Food Regulations (MAFF, 1980) "either expressly or by implication" in a label or advertisement unless "the food is marked or labelled with an indication of the particular aspect of its composition or manufacturing process that gives the food its particular nutritional characteristics" and, if the food has been specially made for the class of person concerned, in addition "the food is marked and labelled with an energy statement". An energy statement is defined, for high energy foods, as a statement of:

"...

(i)   the energy value, expressed in kilojoules and kilocalories, of each hundred grammes or hundred millilitres of the food, as is appropriate, and of a quantified serving of the food, and

(ii) the amount of carbohydrate, protein and fat contained in each hundred grammes or hundred millilitres of the food, as is appropriate, and in a quantified serving of the food...."

For low energy foods, the energy statement must also include "a statement that the energy value of the food is less than 50 kilojoules (12 kilocalories) per hundred grammes or hundred millilitres, as is appropriate."

Thus, alone among those who might wish to give nutritional advice to the public, the food manufacturer is in some circumstances debarred from doing so without publishing the precise facts on which the advice is based. A manufacturer cannot say "eat my product because it has special nutritional qualities which you need" without including on the label a relevant compositional analysis of the product in a most specific form. Any member of the public, on the other hand, however ill-informed, can perfectly legally advise the world in general not to eat the same product for any reason they like to invent—and the manufacturer has no redress.

Many people will remember the recent fulminations of the Director-General of the Health Education Council against the British sliced white loaf. The food manufacturer, if he wished to put the opposite point of view in a label or advertisement, would by law have to support it by scientific data.

It would not be right to draw from the labelling regulations the conclusion that the government does not find the food industry sufficiently responsible to refrain from making unjustified claims for its products, or that the fear that somebody might make an unjustified profit is behind the government's attitude. The thinking is rather that wording on a label can have a direct and effective influence on a consumer at the point of sale or in the home, and so must be strictly controlled; whereas the public bleatings of self-publicists are remote from consumption decisions. Nevertheless the contrast between the treatment of the advice given from the two sources is striking.

On the other hand there is no government control over exhortations to the public to eat this or that provided that no nutritional advantage is claimed if the exhortation is heeded. "Eat more kippers" is a legitimate advertising slogan, "Eat more kippers and keep fit" is probably not. "Eat more X-brand kippers" is probably acceptable, but "Eat more X-brand kippers—the best" is probably not, since it implies that Brand X has qualities which are not found in other brands. The overall law is still in the making, and there will be many court decisions before the legal parameters of what the regulations call "a misleading claim" are fully defined. A veritable sub-culture of labelling expertise is appearing, the exponents of which will argue interminably about the difference in meaning between "flavour" and "flavoured" or how thick a chocolate coating has to be before a biscuit can be described as "thickly coated with chocolate". There is universal agreement that statements on labels and in advertisements should not mislead; there are arguments verging on the metaphysical as to what does or might give a misleading impression.

In all this tangle, there is one saving grace; British civil servants have not lost their sense of humour. Claims in advertisements which are clearly so exaggerated as to be intended to be humorous will not be barred. Nobody will maintain that a beer which is claimed to reach the parts that other beers cannot reach is thereby being advanced as a valuable nutritional beverage with highly specific qualities; and the stirring adventures of young heroes taking boxes of chocolates to the ladies of their dreams will continue to grace our television screens. The reasonable person in Britain is still expected to be able to smile.

Nutrition education

We have thus established that food manufacturers are encouraged, and in many instances compelled, to provide for the consumers the maximum of information about content on the labels of products, and that, if manufacturers seek to amplify that information by indicating that the product may in some way be beneficial, then they become at once subject to additional regulations requiring them to give a scientific analysis of the product so that their customers may—if they are able—judge for themselves whether the claim is justified. The key words are of course "if they are able" and the question raised in the title of this paper is whether, given the requirement for, say, an energy statement to support a nutritional claim on a label, it is the role, or perhaps the responsibility, of the food industry to ensure that the people for whom the statement is provided by law are well-enough informed or sufficiently educated to be able to interpret it, and to understand its implications for the overall diet of themselves and their families.

Let us first agree on the difference between information and education. To inform is to bring facts to somebody's attention. To educate is to give systematic instruction. The giving of information is clearly an important facet of education but education has many other components, one of the essentials being a programme or plan over a considerable period. The difference is that between telling and teaching. To tell a schoolchild that *mensa* is the Latin for table is information. To teach that child Latin is education.

Should, then, the food industry's obligation to inform be extended into an obligation, or at least a desideratum, to educate? The instinctive answer is that it should not. Industrialists are not educators, and above all are not objective as between their own products and those of their competitors—and all food products can be said to be in competition with all other food products, even if it is only in respect of the housekeeping money. Even when industrialists choose to employ skilled educators in the nutritional field, they find difficulty in deciding what they should teach. The greatest admirer of the highly distinguished experts who lead the nutritionist profession could not claim that their doctrines are consistent, either from one person to the next or from one decade to the next. It is tempting for the layperson to reach the conclusion that—to coin a phrase—"one man's meat is another man's poison" and that we who are lucky enough to live in a country where the worst nutritional disorder is obesity should, and can, by trial and error, discover the regime which best suits our individual metabolism, way of life, general health and—perhaps not the least important—enjoyment. Living is a risk business and every day each of us must assess the risks against the advantages of a given course of action. Family shoppers will, even if perfectly aware that eminent nutritionists see dangers in cream buns, nevertheless buy them for their children if they know that they will give great pleasure. Beer drinkers do not consider the nutritional consequences when they order their third pint.

Apart from uncertainty as to what the manufacturer should arrange to be taught or contribute to the curriculum, which would neither be challenged by some nutritionists nor be soon out of date and discredited—who would have thought ten years ago that it would now be respectable to advocate potatoes for health?—the manufacturer faces another difficulty. How can nutritional education be combined with effective propaganda for a manufacturer's own products without denigrating the foods which provide their main competition? By and large the more one eats of one product, the less one eats of another. Can it then be said to be ethical to combine with apparently objective nutritional advice efforts to persuade the reader to eat an individual food?

Those firms which have boldly chosen to enter the field of nutritional education via booklets for teachers and students have chosen different ways of meeting these difficulties. Some make general statements of good nutritional practice in the first half of their booklet and devote the second half to recipes suitable for various categories of consumer, and various occasions, with their own products figuring prominently and by name in those recipes. Some confine their booklets or leaflets to purely objective statements, and do not specify their own products in their recipes, relying simply on the printing of the company name prominently on the covers in order to make the association in the student's mind between that company and good nutritional practice. Some take an altogether different approach and associate themselves with nutritional education by sponsoring and giving their names to seminars, or individual lectures by leading nutritionists, thus performing a public service and also associating their name with highly reputable advice.

The recent trend, however, has been for sectors of the food industry to form organizations whose chief object is to promote the sales of a commodity and products made from it, e.g. the Butter Information Council and the Flour Advisory Bureau. Among their tasks most of these have included the defence of their commodity against attacks, usually on nutritional grounds, and this defence has often been converted into counter-attack, also on nutritional grounds. The virtues and benefits of one's own commodity are emphasized, sometimes perhaps disproportionately, in literature intended to educate; and any opinion or statement critical of that commodity by no matter how distinguished a nutritionist, doctor, other scientist or researcher is countered by quoting the view of a second expert who has reached precisely the opposite conclusion. Since under-nutrition is almost unknown in this country and since medical theories on nutritional matters must therefore wait for years or even generations before they can be proved or disproved, a conflict of view based on genuine belief can nearly always be found. Such quotations as "We cannot begin to achieve true understanding until we forsake our parochial notion that dental caries is the direct outcome of a simple surface battle between acid and enamel..." and "...a biased view of research findings is presented to the public, first by some doctors and second by organizations marketing competitive foods who stand to gain if a certain point of view is generally accepted" abound in this literature, and without presuming to judge the merits and desirability of public mutual recrimination, I would submit that the net result is to confuse the student and not to advance the cause of nutrition education. Teaching must be based on facts, and theories should always be identified as not-proven. I would hazard a guess that most students of home economics and nutrition in this country today are ignorant or confused as to whether saturated or poly-unsaturated fats, if either, are more advisable in the normal person's diet. If they were taught that there were differences of view on the matter — well and good; but I fear that theories have been presented as dogma, and contradicted by counter-dogma; and education has suffered.

Role of the food manufacturing industry

Is there then a role for the food manufacturing industry in nutrition education and, if so, how should that role be played? There is, I am sure, no question of the industry having a responsibility in this field, other than strict adherence to the laws and regulations which I have outlined. The responsibility of the industry is to process safely, to label accurately and to inform fully; beyond these it accepts the task of putting on the shelves the greatest possible variety of manufactured foodstuffs so that the consumer can choose from a maximum range. No manufacturer can know all the factors influencing a single shopper's decisions on a single day—let alone those influencing millions of shoppers on thousands of days: the need to economize, the opportunity to be extravagant, the need to tempt appetites; the knowledge that everybody will be hungry; the various diets of various members of the family; what there is in the larder; who might drop in for a meal; who needs to be spoiled a little, and what it takes—the list is endless and its content cannot be determined. Manufacturers must therefore display their wares so that the controllers of their destinies — the ordinary consumers—can find what they want. And they well know that nutritional elements do not play a very big part in their decisions.

The manufacturers then have, and can have, no responsibility for nutrition education, but can if they wish play a role, and ought to play it well. We have seen some of the difficulties under which they labour if they try to have a hand in education either on their own account or through a trade association of which they are members. By their dedication to the sales of their own products, or to the defence of the safety and excellence of their raw materials, they are tempted to become unobjective and to resort to propaganda rather than education.

Is there then no way in which the food manufacturing industry can play a proper role on the nutrition education scene? Will their contributions always be suspect because of their obvious interest in indicating the merits of their own products and in implying or stating the demerits of the products of their competitors? I believe that there is a way in which the role can be properly played, and which can demonstrate that the public good will override commercial self-interest when motives are suitably harnessed, and the catalyst is the British Nutrition Foundation. It should be no secret that the British Nutrition Foundation is largely the creation of the food manufacturing industry, nor that its scientific and educational work is directed and controlled by committees of eminent scientists whose objectivity has never been challenged. Its role is to provide information, to promote education and to encourage research in food and nutrition with the object of formulating a balanced judgement on nutritional matters. In my view there can be no better way for the industry to play its part in nutritional education than by giving its full support, both financially and morally, to the foundation, and by aiding it in its search after the truth.

One final word. Each manufacturer will of course seek to maximize the sales of their own products and will advertise those products as effectively and widely as possible. Would not the greatest possible contribution from the manufacturers to nutrition education be an agreement that there should be incorporated into advertisements for processed foods a phrase to the effect that all food should be eaten within the framework of a balanced diet, and that prospective customers for the product advertised should take this necessity into account? The need for a balanced diet for ordinary healthy people would seem to be a nutritional imperative with which nobody disagrees. Let the food industry therefore play its part in burning the phrase "balanced diet" into the minds of the people and thus make a more important contribution to nutritional education than it could by any other means.

References

European Council Directive 77/94/EEC on the approximation of the laws of the Member States relating to foodstuffs for particular nutritional uses.

European Council Directive 79/112/EEC on the approximation of the laws of the Member States relating to the labelling, presentation and advertising of foodstuffs to the ultimate consumer.

Food and Drugs Act (1955).

MAFF (January 1980) Proposals for New Labelling of Food Regulations.

Index